EVERYDAY BICYCLING

How to ride a bike for transportation
(whatever your lifestyle)

W0009514

ELLY BLUE

Everyday Bicycling
How to ride a bike for transportation
(whatever your lifestyle)

by Elly Blue

Released December 1, 2012
First printing
ISBN 9781621067252
Cantankerous Titles #18

Cover by Joe Biel
Fonts by Ian Lynam
Designed and Illustrated by Joe Biel
Except illustrations on pages 53, 54, 58 by Ian Lynam
Edited by Joe Biel

Distributed by IPG + Turnaround (UK)

Cantankerous Titles
PO Box 14332
Portland, OR 97293
cantankeroustitles.com
microcosmpublishing.com

Contents

I started riding a bike at age 20. I didn't have a car and wanted a way to get to work that was faster than taking the bus or walking. So I dusted off the barely-used purple three-speed bicycle that had been too large for me as a child and started to ride.

Bicycling was a revelation. I felt free when I rode. I could do more and see more in a day than ever before. But it was also a learning process. At first, I rode everywhere on the sidewalk. I had weekly wardrobe malfunctions until I learned to roll up my right pants leg and ditched my pencil skirts and tight jackets. I ran through red lights without a thought, and had some close calls. My purse straps dangled through the bottom of my front basket and got caught in my spokes. Riding without fenders in the winter, I went everywhere with a stripe of mud up the back of my coat.

I only learned to ride a bike confidently and safely several years later, after I moved to Portland, Oregon. I made friends with other people who rode bikes everywhere and who loved to talk over every minute detail of cycling. I loved it. From them, I learned to ride in the street in a straight line, to be cautious at intersections, and how and when to signal and yield and merge. I bought lights and fenders and tools and a u-lock and started wearing a helmet. I traded in my heavy old three-speed cruiser for a mountain bike with racks and panniers and found I could carry anything I needed. My proudest moment was when a friend gave me a television and I brought it home on my bike. I stopped asking friends with cars for rides and started riding longer distances just for fun.

Now, 15 years after I began, riding a bicycle is second nature. It can be difficult to remember that I didn't always know the things that now seem like common sense, like making sure my bungie cords stay out of my wheels and never passing another cyclist on the right. Seeing the huge growth of new riders in Portland and the rest of the country in the last few years has brought back those early memories and inspired me to write this book.

Bicycling is fun, safe, and easier and faster than any other mode of transportation. It saves me money, makes me healthy, and above all it brings me joy every day. I learned everything that makes all this possible from the other people riding bikes around me, and am still learning. I want to pass along some of this knowledge to you.

This book is a resource for people who are new to bicycle transportation as well as for those who are looking to make their everyday bicycling experience more awesome.

My hope is that this book will inspire you with the confidence and curiosity to continue asking questions and trying new things as you pursue the pleasure of exploring your world by bicycle.

Enjoy the ride!

—Elly Blue, Portland, Oregon, July 2012
everydaybicycling.com

Bicycling for transportation has become hugely popular in recent years. Many thousands of people are taking up cycling, each of them with a unique set of reasons. People ride for fitness, for fashion, to save money, to save time, for environmental reasons, out of political motivations (on both sides of the aisle), to spend time with friends and family, to remember what it felt like to be young, or simply for the joy of it.

If you've made the decision to start riding, or have an inkling that you might, you've come to the right place. This book is intended to help you integrate bicycling into your daily life in a way that works for you, no matter what your reasons for riding.

You often hear people say, in a self-deprecating tone, "I'm just a fair weather cyclist," or "I only ride on weekends." But any time you get on a bike, that's great. It doesn't matter if you drive or take transit for nine months of the year, or put your bike on the car and drive halfway to work and ride the rest of the way, or keep your riding strictly to your neighborhood. Any time you ride a bike, that's more than enough.

All you need to get started bicycling is the bike itself and the will to ride it. But bicycling often becomes easier and more fun when you have people to talk about all the details with. This book is no replacement for those friends, but it's a start—a set of ideas and resources to try out, debate, and decide on for yourself.

You will at times encounter people who have strong, and often loud, opinions about every aspect of how you ride. Some of these folks will have been riding longer than you, some will have written books or blogs, some will be industry professionals, and some will just be eager to speak their mind. Listen to them if you like, but don't let their opinions and theories override your own experience, knowledge, and needs.

Most bicycle transportation guides are written for people whose only needs are commuting to and from work. But for most of us, our transportation needs are more complicated than that. This book should demonstrate that a bicycle is more than capable of rising to most any challenge.

Let's start by looking at the very basic things you need to know about operating a bicycle on the road. Then we'll help you integrate these bicycling skills into your daily life, choose the right bicycle, and keep it in good working order. My favorite topic follows: how to carry anything by bicycle (yes, anything!). Later on in the book I turned to the growing community of families who get around by bike to cover the ins and outs of bicycling with children. And the final chapter is for those who want to improve their communities for cycling, be it through whimsical fun or political advocacy.

Whatever your reasons, style, and experiences riding, don't forget to have fun!

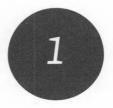

How to ride a bike

So you've decided to give bicycling a try. Congratulations!

It's easy. It's fun! You just get on the bike and ride.

Right?

Well, sort of.

That's all I knew when I first started riding around town. I wasn't the greatest bike rider, poking along on the sidewalk to the dismay of people trying to walk there. Sometimes I'd get in the street, but I wouldn't always slow down or look first. And I wasn't always very steady on the bicycle. One time, I turned my head towards a distant sound and ended up riding into a wall. On another occasion I was standing at a red light, waiting, and just fell down in a heap with my bike on top of me.

It was only years later, when I joined an email list for detailed discussions about all the minutiae of riding in traffic that I learned how much I didn't know. As I made more friends who also rode everywhere, we talked about what we were doing, what gear we used, what routes we chose, how to be part of traffic.

Once I began to learn, my transition from wobbly novice to confident everyday rider was only a matter of time. I hope this chapter can serve to let you in on some of the basics I wish someone had told me back in 1999.

Learning to ride

If your last time on a bike was as a kid, getting back in the saddle might be just like riding a bike—or it might not be so pat.

Starting from scratch

The most difficult part of learning to ride, hands down, will be walking out the door with your bike. Take a deep breath. You can do it!

The best place to learn is a quiet back street or an empty parking lot. Lower your bike seat all the way so that you can put your feet on the ground while you sit. Scoot around, lifting your feet off the ground and coasting for longer each time. Have a friend hold on or guide you at first if it helps. But eventually, they'll need to let go. It's counterintuitive, but the faster you go, the easier it will be to balance.

Starting and stopping can be tricky at first. Think of your pedal as a step for climbing up and down to the seat. Think about where you will want your pedals to be when you start again, and plan accordingly. On most bikes you can turn your pedals backwards while you're stopped to get them positioned for a strong start.

Try to anticipate stops in advance so you can brake slowly, using both hands at once. The rear brake should be your default when you're first learning. The front brake will stop you faster and better, but if you grab it hard by itself you risk locking up your front wheel and flying head-first over your handlebars.

Until you develop an instinct for the bike, your body will want to steer it in whatever direction you are looking. While you're still in the parking lot, practice riding in as straight a line as possible while looking left and right and glancing back over each shoulder.

Your skill, experience, and fitness aren't important. The main things you need are patience and confidence. If the person helping you learn is making you feel anxious or self-conscious, ditch them. It's time for you to learn how to fly!

Each new thing will feel a little clumsy the first few times you do it. After that, you'll never think about it again. It might take only ten minutes to learn to ride. It might take an hour. It might take several sessions in the parking lot. You may not get everything right away, but keep going and you'll master the art of bicycling faster than you can believe.

Advanced road skills
Riding a bicycle is amazingly simple, yet there is always more to learn. If you've already mastered the art of staying upright in the saddle, but wish for the skills and confidence to handle every situation in traffic, it's worth continuing your education.

In most cities, you'll find a handful of League Certified Instructors (LCIs), trained by the League of American Bicyclists to teach adults and youth to ride safely in traffic, through a series of day long classes. If League instruction is not available, the motorcycle training course offered by your local DMV can be an invaluable opportunity to learn defensive two-wheeled driving.

For those who prefer to learn on their own, the two classic guides to advanced transportation cycling skills are *Effective Cycling* by John Forester and *The Art of Cycling* by Robert Hurst.

Hitting the road

No matter what your level of experience with riding, starting out biking in traffic for the first time will seem new and strange. The good news, though, is how quickly it becomes second nature. Truly anyone can ride a bicycle. You'll learn best as you ride; in the meantime, here are some basic ideas to build on and make your own.

Being traffic

Here are three maxims for riding a bicycle on the road: Put safety first, for yourself and others. Be courteous second. Third, be legal.

The thing to keep in mind about traffic is that it isn't just cars. When you're on a bicycle, you are not just navigating traffic: You are a part of traffic. So is everyone else in the roadway, whether they're biking, driving, walking, skateboarding, running to catch their bus, getting out of a car, or standing on the corner waiting to cross. Even if someone is not behaving legally and predictably, they are still traffic.

Your job is to pay attention. Notice who has the right of way at each moment. Yield or move forward when it's your turn. Be constantly alert for exceptions, like when someone cuts in front of you and you need to yield out of turn. Sometimes this will mean you'll need to act just like you're driving; sometimes you'll act like a pedestrian; all the time you'll be on a bike.

Not everyone will agree with everything written here. And not everything will apply to every person or every city or every road. Take it all with a grain of salt. Think about it, talk about it, and err on the side of caution when you can. Whatever you do, ride predictably, communicate clearly, and pay attention. So long as you remember that everyone else on the road may not be doing these things, you'll be okay.

Choosing a route

Most people, when they first start riding, choose by instinct to ride on the most direct route to where they're going, the same one you take while driving or on the bus.

The problem with the most direct route is that it's likely to be a fast arterial road that goes straight from your house to your destination. But by all means, if you can ride comfortably on it, go for it. Use this chapter as your guide for how to handle yourself.

Most people don't love these roads. They are fast, they are loud, they reek of exhaust, and people in cars don't always expect to see you there and may express that aggressively. If there's a bike lane on this road, it may just be your best bet—but be cautious of those turning cars.

To find other routes, your best friend is a map. If your area has a bike map, you may be able to get one for free from the transportation department or a bike shop. If there is no bike map, then find the most detailed street map you can and look for different ways to go.

If you know someone else who rides, talk with them about which roads they like best and least. There might be a detour that takes you through quiet, residential streets, trading an extra ten minutes of travel time for your sanity.

Once you start trying out every permutation of how to get from point A to point B, you'll soon find your favorite ways, as well as the fastest. You may end up needing to get creative. The trickiest parts of the route will doubtless be the crossings of busy streets. Sometimes these will require you to make yet another detour, or to get off your bike and act like a pedestrian, or to ride on the sidewalk for half a block. You probably aren't the only person who has trouble with these difficult connections. See Chapter 6 for advocacy tips.

Don't be a salmon

"[There is] a group of riders who are a menace to us all. I am referring of course to those directionally-challenged irritants known as 'bike salmon.'"
—BikeSnobNYC

Always ride with traffic, not against it.

This advice may go against what you learned as a kid. Conventional wisdom used to be to always walk and bike facing traffic, so you could see what was coming and get out of the way. But that advice, like so many childhood myths, turns out to be not just wrong, but more dangerous.

Wrong way cyclists are more likely to get into a crash than people riding with traffic. Why? In a word: Intersections. And one more word: Driveways. And parking lot exits. People in cars look left before they turn right, because that's where they expect traffic—including you—to be coming from.

If you live in a city with a lot of one-way streets, it's tempting to ride the wrong way down them as an alternative to riding three blocks around. Some cities are starting to see the wisdom of converting one way streets back to two directions, in part to accommodate this natural flow.

I don't advise wrong way riding for any reason. Nobody expects to see you coming, and police love to write tickets for this.

Neighborhood streets

Quiet neighborhood streets are often the best places to ride. Car traffic is relatively slow, there's more room to share than on a separated path, and you have yards and houses to look at and people to say hello to.

Even on neighborhood streets, it's a good idea to take the lane. Ride in a relatively straight line, without weaving in and out of the spaces between parked cars. Keep a nice, car-door length buffer between yourself and any parked cars. Keep your eyes open for people doing neighborhoody things like backing out of a driveway or running into the street. And be extra cautious at intersections; many drivers take a casual approach to stop signs on neighborhood streets. You need to be at least as alert for cross-traffic at intersections where you have the right of way as at ones where you don't.

Bike lanes

Bike lanes, while they are a beautiful thing, don't guarantee your safety, and aren't always well-designed. Often, the bike lane puts you in the direct path of opening car doors, turning cars and trucks, wrong-way cyclists, pedestrians stepping out from between parked cars, and other hazards.

On many busy streets, having a bike lane is much better than having no bike lane at all—it reminds drivers that you have the right to be on the road, and carves out a small space for you to occupy. Whenever you are in a bike lane, stay alert and be prepared to stop or merge at a moment's notice.

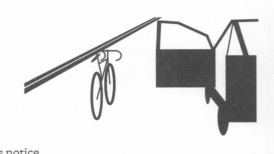

Busy streets

When you're riding on a street without a bike lane, or if the bike lane is full of gravel or glass, where do you belong in the traffic lane?

Riding rght down the middle of it.

This is daunting, but important.

Many new riders will instinctively hug the edge of the road, no matter how narrow it is. When there's an intersection or a space between parked cars, it's tempting to weave to the right to buy a momentary sense of breathing room before plunging back into the fray.

Similarly, the main reason it's a bad idea to ride in the parking lane is the danger of not being seen by the people driving behind you or turning onto the road in front of you.

In fact, the safest place to ride in a narrow traffic lane is nearly always far enough to the left to put you, if there are parked cars, at least four feet from the line of parked cars—safely out of the danger of getting knocked off your bike when someone suddenly flings open their car door in your path.

It's a good idea to ride towards the center of the lane even if there are no parked cars. There is a psychological reason for this. When you ride further to the left, your position signals to people driving behind you that it is not safe to pass you in the same lane; they are more likely to fully merge, giving you enough space, or else wait until it's safe to pass. Riding all the way to the right, on the other hand, tempts the person behind you to squeeze past, dangerously close.

On the other hand, when there are people behind you who want to pass and you actually do have space to move over—for instance, an entire block with no parked cars—treat it as any other lane merge. Check over your shoulder, signal that you'll be moving right, and then move right. Be sure to give yourself enough space to merge back left into the travel lane when your window ends, and do it properly, with a look and a signal.

People may need to wait a minute to pass you, it's true, and some people will get impatient. It's okay. They can pass in the next lane when they have an opening, or when it's safe for you to pull to the right. If the person behind you is not slowing down, or if an impatient line of cars is building up, you can always pull over and let them by. And while I don't recommend weaving between lanes, sometimes riding with a little bit of a wiggle can signal to the drivers behind you that they need to give you some extra room when they do pass you.

Taking the lane applies on busy and quiet streets alike. Practice on the quiet ones first, the ones where you are probably going the speed of car traffic anyway. It might feel strange at first, but you'll find that you feel more confident and that people in cars give you more breathing room and act more predictably as well.

If you have a wide shoulder available, then by all means use it. And if there is a lot of aggressive traffic with speeds greater than 25 or 30 mph, it's probably better to find another route. Otherwise, take that lane.

Sidewalks
In some places it is illegal to ride on the sidewalk, and in others it is the only reasonable place. But you're almost always better off in the street, even if it means taking an alternate route. Your chances of being hit on the sidewalk by someone turning in or out of a driveway are higher than if you are in the street. And you also pose a danger to people walking or stepping out of doorways.

If you must ride on the sidewalk, then behave as much like a pedestrian as possible. Ride at the speed of a walk or a slow jog; be alert and prepared to stop at any time. Be most careful at intersections. Stop and look both ways before crossing.

Sharing the path

Off-road paths, rail trails, multi-use paths, linear parks—whatever you call them, they're paved trails, usually along waterfronts or disused rail lines. Originally intended for recreation, they're coming to serve as important bicycle transportation links. On any given day, you'll find people bicycling, walking, jogging, rollerblading, and pushing strollers, often with kids and dogs. Unfortunately, this mix is not always compatible on an eight or twelve foot wide path.

When many people first start to ride a bike, they feel most comfortable on these paths, away from car traffic. They can be quite safe, especially if they are relatively empty of other traffic; but when paths like these are crowded they are the site of a relatively high number of crashes. Just like on the road, you cannot have any expectation of how your fellow path users will behave in any given situation.

You can ride on these paths relatively safely if you treat them with appropriate caution. If nobody's in sight and there are no intersections, go as fast as you want. When you need to pass someone, slow down—to their speed if necessary, and stopping if necessary. Give them ample space as you pass and an audible warning well before. Assume they are just as likely to swerve out in front of you as to move over. Likewise, be alert to the possibility of someone passing you, and try not to weave and swerve, or ride side-by-side on a crowded path.

Intersections

Intersections are where most crashes happen. When you're bicycling, it's important to be hyperaware and to remember that people turning—left or right—probably will not see you, especially if you are all the way to the right, or if it's pouring down rain. It's also important not to rely on people's turn signals or lack thereof. Eye contact, on the other hand, is an excellent tool. Here's a run down on how to handle yourself at intersections.

Turning

Signal your turns!

Signaling is traditionally done with the left arm. Hold it out straight to signal a left turn, up at 90 degrees to signal a right turn, and down at 90 degrees to show your intention to stop or slow down.

You can also signal a right turn by holding your right arm out straight. This method is subject to debate. Proponents point out that it makes more sense to drivers, many of whom have forgotten their long-ago driver's ed classes and interpret the traditional right turn signal to mean you're waving hello (or worse). Opponents say that you're better off having a hand by your right (rear) brake in case you need to stop suddenly. Whichever you choose, always signal your turns!

Left turns off of busy roads can pose a sticky situation, since you're most likely to be over to the right. Sometimes you're even required to be on the right. So how do you turn left?

You have a couple of options. You can turn just as though you were in a car, signaling, looking over your shoulder, and merging left in the block before your turn.

If traffic is fast or you'd just rather stay to the right, or in the bike lane, you can also avail yourself of the practice known as the "Copenhagen left." Stay to the right as you go through the intersection, being wary as always of turning cars. Stop at the opposite corner. Make sure you're out of the path of whoever is behind you and turn your bike 90 degrees so you are facing the

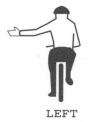

LEFT

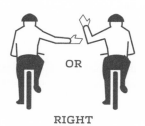

OR

RIGHT

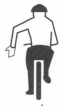

SLOW/STOP

direction you want to go. When that light turns green, voila, you're ready to continue ahead.

The art of yielding

Yielding is a constant question. Who has the right of way? Who goes first?

According to the letter of the law, you should yield the same exact way on a bike as you should in a car. There are exceptions in some states, but for the most part this holds true.

If you have a stop sign, yield. If you have a red light, yield. When in doubt, yield to whoever is on your right. Yield to anyone who is in front of you. Yield to the bus. Always, always, always yield to pedestrians, schoolbuses, and emergency vehicles.

At a four way stop or an intersection without stop signs, the person who gets there first gets to go first. If two people arrive at the same time, the person to the right goes first. If someone is waiting to cross the street, smile and wave them across.

Be confident in asserting your right of way. But even when you don't have to, sometimes it's best to yield anyway. If someone's clearly in a hurry, or you're concerned they might not see you, let them go first. Give some extra leeway to anyone who is clearly confused or impaired. In all cases, do what's safe and polite, and be ready to correct your course when things change.

In a car, the culture is all about racing up and claiming your right of way. On a bicycle, it's all too tempting to behave the same way. But you have more to lose on a bike—and more to gain. On a bike, yield your right of way with generosity rather than aggression.

To stop or not to stop

Ah yes. Stopping. In any conversation about bicycling, no subject except helmets is guaranteed to raise more heated opinions.

Some say absolute compliance with the law is the only option. Others retort that there's a double standard and that most people don't come to a complete stop while driving. Yet others argue that bicycling is different enough from driving that the same laws don't make sense.

When it comes to actual situations on the road, these arguments quickly break down. The strict legalist rolls, slowly and cautiously, through the stop sign. The avowed rebels might wait for the light to change even when nobody is coming. Here's a guide to how to handle the situation on the ground.

Red lights

Red lights provide the clearest guidance for everyone. When the light is green, go. When it is red or yellow, stop.

Easy, right? But there's a catch. In many places, red lights are programmed to only turn green when a car shows up. So what happens when you're waiting and waiting....but there's no car?

This was the dilemma that led Idaho, in 1981, to pass legislation allowing people on bicycles to go forward if the way was clear after stopping at a red light. The law was deemed preferable to the expense of retrofitting every major intersection in the state to detect bicycles.

If your local lights can be triggered by a bicycle, then learn the trick of doing this. Usually there is a metal circle or diamond on the ground. If you position one of your wheels to touch part of it, the metal of your spokes and rims should trigger the light to change. If they aren't set up this way, then you have a dilemma. One option is to go forward, Idaho style, as soon as it's safe, treating the light as though it were a stop sign. In some places, the law allows this. In others it doesn't, in which case you may be better off dismounting your bike to cross like a pedestrian.

Stop signs

Stop signs pose their own set of questions. The other famous component of the Idaho stop law is a clause that allows people on bicycles to treat stop signs as though they are yield signs.

Yielding does not mean blowing through at full speed. Think of the Idaho stop as what a runner would do before crossing a street. It means slowing down to nearly a stop and looking left, then right, then left again to make sure the coast is clear. If it isn't, stop. If it is, proceed with caution.

The Idaho stop, though not legally sanctioned in any of the other 49 states, is a nearly universal practice among bicycle riders. Even when done safely, it has significant downsides. Where there is police enforcement around stop signs, fines are often very high. If running a stop sign causes a crash, any resulting court case or insurance decision will not likely go well for you. For many reasons including these, I recommend riding safely and yielding when appropriate at all times.

Other situations
Road rage
It will happen. Someone will swerve too close or shout at you to get off the road. You'll experience an adrenaline rush, and some combination of fear and anger.

It's easy to rage back. But tempting as it may be to return fire with a middle finger or a few choice insults, it's often far better not to escalate an argument with someone of unknown temper who is driving a two ton vehicle. Let the moment go and continue on your way.

Seize the opportunity to practice memorizing license plate numbers. If the person was obviously drunk, or if they hit you or threw something at you, call 911. You have the right to ride down the street without being threatened, assaulted, or harassed.

The zen of bicycling
You can notice a lot from the seat of the bike; you see the world from new angles. But at the same time, it's all too easy to get distracted from the sights and sounds and smells around you. Bicycling is an opportunity to practice existing in the moment, noticing your breath, your bicycle, and everything around you. You'll enjoy yourself, ride more safely, and be less prone to road rage.

What to do if you are in a crash

If you are involved in a crash, or witness one, call 911 immediately. Get the car's license plate number and the driver's insurance information, if possible. Make sure you get contact information for any witnesses. Call the police and insist on a report. If you might be injured, get it looked at even if you don't feel hurt in the adrenaline spike of the moment. Write down every detail you can recall before you sleep.

If the other person has insurance, it should cover your medical and bike repair or replacement costs. If you have car insurance, that should also cover you in the same way while you're on your bicycle. If neither you nor the other person has car insurance, your own health insurance, if you have it, may cover your bills, and your homeowner's or renter's insurance may cover your bike. Begin the saga of dealing with insurance right away.

If your bike is damaged, you'll need to have it evaluated by a bike shop in order for insurance to cover repair or replacement. Different bike shops will give wildly different assessments of the same bike, so it's worth going to two or three.

Bicycle crashes occupy a grey area in bureaucratic procedures. Your situation may not be a perfect fit with the paperwork someone has in front of them, and this can tempt people to cut corners or skip over your case. It's unfortunate, but in many places police, media, insurance adjustors, and juries will empathize with the motorist and assume that the person riding the bicycle was at fault, no matter what actually happened. Insist on being treated fairly, double check every detail, and when in doubt get a lawyer—preferably one who rides a bike herself.

Outfitting yourself for safety

You can help make your presence and intentions on the road clear by the way you ride; you can make it even more clear by making yourself as visible and audible as possible.

Visibility

You may have seen her, perhaps just at the last minute—the cycling ninja, riding down an unlit residential street at night, in all black, with no lights, perhaps taking a far-too-casual approach to stop signs.

While it's true that there are no guarantees when it comes to safety, on or off the bike, it can only help to make yourself more visible.

You don't have to spend a lot of money or adhere to a certain look. The one key is, as with everything, to do what you feel comfortable with and what works with your lifestyle and budget.

Make a more informed decision by having a friend put on something similar to the setup you use and ride around the block in the dark. If they aren't clearly visible from half a block away, then adjust what you're doing until it works.

Lights

In the U.S., most bicycles do not come with lights. Yet in most states you are required to have lights on your bike at night or in dark weather. Specifics vary widely—it's a good idea to look up your local statute.

Law aside, you will definitely need a front light (usually white) and a rear light (usually red).

Beyond that, the type of light you need depends largely on where you ride at night. If you are primarily on well-lit city streets, then your main goal is to be seen. If your commute takes you along unmaintained roads or unlit paths, then you'll want a headlight that will illuminate the road ahead of you.

Prices range from $5 for little rubber lights that run on watch batteries to hundreds of dollars for what amounts to spotlights. If your comfort level and budget tend towards the latter, be aware of oncoming traffic and turn the beam slightly downward so that you don't blind people.

The most common variety of lights are small, battery powered "blinkies" that clip on to mounts that you can attach to your handlebars and seat post. A cheap set of these are good starter lights, though they tend to break, their mounts are annoying, and they tend to get turned on in your bag and run out of batteries at the most inconvenient times.

If you leave these lights on your bike, they will eventually be stolen. I generally clip a red blinkie onto my waistband or bag rather than the bike itself so that I don't forget to take it off when I park. The front light goes on your handlebars and is easier to remember. Some people like to attach their lights to their helmets with rubber bands or special mounts. Others hedge their bets with two sets of lights with staggered battery life—one for the bike, one for the helmet.

If you're stranded on a dark night with only one set of working batteries, the front light is your best choice for them. People driving up behind you can still see you in their headlights if you have no rear light, especially if you have a reflector back there. Your greatest danger comes from people turning off of side streets in front of you. Their headlights are pointed away from you, further up the road, making it difficult for them to see you coming.

Generator lights

Battery-powered lights are quick and easy and can be cheap. Grab some and start riding! But for the long run, plan on getting yourself free of them.

Generator lights mount permanently to your bike, are difficult to steal, and will never be forgotten or run out of batteries. Standard 60 years ago, today they're coming back into style as more people want the convenience of just being able to get on the bike and go.

Friction generators are the classics. A little roller rests against your tire and powers your light when your wheel turns. You push a lever to release the roller when it's daylight. As you can guess, this type of light will slow you down a bit, creating marginally more work as you pedal.

Hub generator lights are the more modern solution. They run off the energy produced by moving parts inside your wheel as it turns, not slowing you down one bit. You will need to buy a new wheel for each light, so these are a substantial investment.

Another type of light is powered by magnets that you clip to your spokes. Each time a magnet passes the light it gets a small burst of power, just enough to flash (many cycle computers work the same way). Some models have a battery built in that can hold a charge for a few minutes so that your lights continue to flash while you are stopped at a light. Magnet lights have the disadvantage of being fairly dim and low to the ground, but are excellent in better-lit areas or if you like to run two sets of lights. They are a value at $45 to $60 per set with no need to buy batteries.

Get reflective

I used to scoff at reflectors and reflective gear—until one night when I accepted a ride home from a friend. We drove slowly up a road with a heavily trafficked bike lane on the right. The reflective panels on the backs of panniers, jackets, and shoes, nearly invisible by day, glowed like a beacon in our headlights, far outshining the firefly flickering of battery-powered blinkies.

In some places, a red rear reflector is a legal alternative to a red rear light. It's good to have one even if you ride with a light—it will never run out of batteries or get stolen or wiggle its way off your waistband to break open on the ground.

Many new bikes and most older ones come equipped with reflectors on the seatpost, on the headtube, on the pedals, and in the spokes. If your bike doesn't have these, look for cheap reflectors in the parts bin at your local bike repair coop, or new ones for sale online.

For better coverage and more creativity, you can buy reflective sticky tape in several colors. Several intrepid companies sell kits with pre-cut reflective tape to cover all parts of your bike, helmet, and gear in various colors and patterns. You can buy little, reflective stickers to adorn your helmet and water bottle that come in shapes ranging from hearts to spaceships. There are even lines of jewelry and clothing made of reflective materials.

Keep in mind that reflectors will make you more visible in a car's headlights—but only lights will enable someone who is walking or bicycling to see you on a dark road.

Clothing

Light colored clothing makes a big difference in being visible at night. As you ride more and your wardrobe evolves, you may find yourself choosing the light green sweater over the dark brown one.

If you want the extra visibility, many technical apparel companies sell jackets so bright yellow they hurt your eyes and show up in headlights like great green flares. There are also many products you can deck yourself out with, from the bright orange safety vest to reflective ankle straps.

Sometimes the best strategy for daytime visibility is to look a little out of the ordinary. In some places this might simply mean wearing a suit and tie or a skirt and heels to ride. In others, a top hat or proverbial clown suit might be what you need to stand out. See Chapter 2 for more on the bicycling wardrobe.

The humble bicycle bell

If you want to be heard by truck drivers, buy an air horn for your handlebars. For other situations, the classic bicycle bell is the ideal tool for letting somebody know that you are coming along the road towards their about-to-open car door, or that are about to pass them on the bike path.

All bikes used to come with bells. Back in the 1950s, bells were a part of the transportation vernacular. People simply knew: if you hear a bike bell, move to the right.

This is a practice worth bringing back. You can buy a bell for your bike at any bike shop for around $5 and mount it to your handlebars in seconds with a screwdriver. If you want something that will make a nicer sound and last more than a year, you'll end up spending $10 or $15.

If you have no bell, saying "on your left" prior to passing someone can be effective but be prepared for it to be misunderstood by a surprised pedestrian whose instinct is to step left when hearing the word "left."

Mirrors

Mirrors that attach to either your helmet or handlebars can be obtained for under $15.

A mirror can help you see what's sneaking up on you—the city bus with the engine in the back that you don't hear until it's breathing down your neck, or fellow bike rider about to recklessly squeeze by you on the right in the bike lane.

For urban riding, you need to constantly be aware of what's happening 360 degrees around you. Some people find mirrors to be distracting in the city and not as useful as a full-on, head-swiveling glance over the shoulder.

But if you spend a lot of time sharing fast, narrow roads with cars that primarily come from one direction—directly behind you—a mirror can be a lifesaver once you've perfected that regular quick little glance.

Helmets

"I began wearing a helmet when I undertook responsibility toward a significant other, not for myself. I have gotten used to it, and it is a very convenient place to hang a mirror." —R.W., Portland

Based on the data available, you would be wise to wear a helmet while riding in a car or walking along or across any busy road. But only when you ride a bicycle are helmets expected and socially acceptable. I wear one almost every time I ride and have been particularly glad of it twice. I recommend that you wear a helmet as well, and that you make sure that it fits over your forehead and that the straps are adjusted properly to keep it in place.

That said, helmets are far from the last word in bicycle safety. Helmets provide limited protection in specific circumstances. They protect you the most in the sort of crashes that typically happen riding at slower speeds and on streets without many cars. In fast traffic, there are more types of crashes that can happen, and helmets will serve you well in some of them.

But in the bigger picture, bicycle helmets have no ability to prevent crashes or create a safer transportation system. In places where helmet use is legally required, fewer people tend to ride bikes—which has the effect of making cycling more dangerous.

A final note on safety

This chapter should give you an idea of how to ride confidently, predictably, and defensively. These practices, plus some alertness and caution, should keep you reasonably safe. Helmets can protect you from certain kinds of crashes, and audible and visual signals can help you communicate your presence and intentions to others.

But the one single thing that's been proven to significantly improve bicycle safety is the presence of more people riding bikes on the road.

That's it. It's no cure-all, but the more people out there on bikes, the more understanding, attention, and respect we tend to get from people driving cars and trucks.

There is recent research showing that this safety in numbers phenomenon is enjoyed not only by people bicycling, but by everyone else on the road. The simple presence of bike lanes on a road has been found to make streets safer for people walking and even driving.

There are no guarantees in life; using the roads, whether you're driving, bicycling, or walking, is the most dangerous thing you'll do on any given day. But safety is not just a matter of what happens in crashes. Research consistently shows that the risks posed to your health by inactivity are far greater than any risks incurred while transporting yourself around by two wheels or two feet.

So get out there and ride. Do the best you can, and don't forget to have fun.

2

Your life, by bike

"It's easier to bike if you have your things organized. If you have your bag and your gloves and your rain cape and your lights all together and you know where they are, you can just grab them and go. If you need to go and you can't find your gloves, you'll be annoyed." —Sara S.

When I started riding a bike, I didn't make any wardrobe changes until I had to. At the time I had a professional office job, so I wore skirts, polyester blouses, and jackets. As I biked, my wardrobe evolved. My tighter skirts tended to split up the seams, sometimes requiring emergency safety-pin repairs at work. The fuller, longer ones would become mangled in the spokes, and I migrated towards trousers and flared, knee-length skirts. Loose, usually cotton blouses replaced sweat-producing (and smelly!) polyester ones. Most of my jackets were too tight across my shoulders when I reached forward for the handlebars, so I took to wearing sweaters instead.

As I biked more and more frequently the less functional clothes got pushed to the back of my closet and eventually out of my life. These changes happened gradually, but eventually all my clothes were far more comfortable and durable, on and off the bike, than what I'd been wearing before.

Your life, by bike

Starting to bike is a bit like getting a new piece of furniture or moving to a new neighborhood. You'll need to rearrange some things and change some habits to make everything functional and harmonious.

When you switch from driving or transit to bicycling, it's like you suddenly have a whole different map of your community. Bicycling changes the pace of your life.

Some trips will be much faster by bike. You won't be stuck in traffic or on the bus, you can take short cuts, and you won't have to look for parking. Bicycling can make your commute time more predictable, and in many cases even faster than driving—particularly when you factor in the vagaries of rush hour traffic and parking. The same 15 mph speed that feels painfully slow in a car can be exhilarating on a bike.

Other trips will be slower. You might be stuck weaving through back streets with stop signs every block rather than taking the direct but dangerous six lane arterial that you're used to driving on. The freeway, instead of making your trip across town magically fast, becomes a barrier that you need to go out of your way to cross.

You might start planning your week's errands in advance, leaving more time between obligations, and shifting your daily travel patterns to shorten distances and reduce the number of trips you take. You'll find you spend a few more minutes gathering your things to leave the house—do you have your lights? Is your water bottle full? Enough air in the tires? Is it glove weather yet?

But slowing down doesn't necessarily mean losing time. If you replace a trip to the gym with a half hour commute each way one day a week, you've just saved both time and money. Pedaling your kids to school in a cargo bike rather than driving them adds up to more quality time spent with your family. A ride in the morning can clear your head and make your day's work more efficient and fruitful.

As your map of the city shifts, so will your life. How fast or slow you want your bicycling life to be is a choice that will help determine what kind of bicycle you ride, what you wear, and even where you work, what you buy, and how you socialize.

Some parts of this will be thrilling, others blissful, others deeply frustrating. Sometimes you'll find you want to ride fast, others slow. Sometimes it's not worth it to bike at all. There's no right and wrong way to do it.

Work

Recently I met a lawyer who told me that she loves to go on recreational bike rides on the weekends. She wanted to start riding the four miles into work once a week, but was concerned about being able to commute by bike while maintaining a professional appearance.

I suggested that she take a trial run on a weekend. That experience would help her figure out her clothes, her bike set-up, how much time it would take, and what to expect on her route. She wrote back the next week and said she'd begun commuting and found it far easier than she had expected—and was having a blast.

Bicycle commuting doesn't have to be complicated—and if your commute is your major transportation need every day, it can be very simple indeed.

Many guides recommend that commuters wear technical bicycling kits with padded shorts, driving once a week to bring a fresh set of clothes to the office. If your commute is longer than five miles or so each way, or if you are commuting in very hot or rainy weather, this might be your best strategy.

Some work places have showers and locker rooms available where bike commuters can clean up and change clothes when they arrive at work. At others, you'll need to manage with a bathroom sink.

For many people, though, all this isn't necessary. Bicycling to work does not have to be an athletic pursuit, and can be done wearing professional attire and carrying all your work things in a pannier, plus a rain jacket and a spare set of dry socks just in case. The wardrobe tips further down in this chapter should help you to maintain the dress code of your workplace while bicycling.

Parking your bicycle while you are at work may be more of a challenge. If you live in a city with relatively low levels of bike theft, parking on the street shouldn't be a problem. Some office buildings have designated bike parking areas or rooms; in some cities this is required, and it's always worth asking. You also may be able to simply bring your bike into your office, perhaps using the freight elevator.

If your workplace is truly not bicycle friendly, it may be necessary to take creative measures, such as investing in a cheap bicycle that can be parked outside all day, or in a folding bicycle that you can keep tucked under your desk.

An increasing number of cities offer commuters centrally located "bike stations" that provide secure, indoor bike parking for a membership fee. These are often located next to transit hubs, and some of them provide locker rooms and even showers for members to use and are attached to full-service bike shops.

Shopping and errands
Commuting to work is hardly the limit of our weekly transportation needs. We must eat, and there are groceries to buy, sometimes in large quantities. There are basic household needs like dish soap, toilet paper. Perhaps you have laundry or dry cleaning to transport. And what about furniture, lumber, plumbing supplies, or a young apple tree? It's possible to carry all of these things and more by bicycle. How to do so is covered thoroughly in the next chapter.

If you are transitioning from driving to bicycling, you may find yourself shopping for groceries and everything else more frequently, buying smaller quantities at a time. This can potentially be more expensive and time consuming than doing big weekly shops at discount stores on the outskirts of town. But it also might end up being surprisingly easier and, in the long run, more affordable.

Others, particularly parents of young children, find that when they start bicycling they shop less often, doing as many errands as possible once a week or less.

As you explore your neighborhood by bike you may end up finding a variety of different options you might not have otherwise noticed. Look for family-owned grocery stores specializing in imported food, corner markets with a decent selection of fresh vegetables, and small stores that sell everything from blank paper to curtain rods to fresh baked bread.

You may find that shopping more frequently and closer to home takes less time than a long weekend outing, and that buying only what you need for the next two days results in less waste. Or you may not—and if you find yourself renting or borrowing a car every week or two to stock up, that's great. It's all about figuring out what works best for you.

Social life

If the people you spend most of your time with don't ride, you may find yourself as a passenger in a car when you are with them—or they may find themselves joining you on a bicycle.

Sometimes things can get awkward. Some people will incessantly ask, with a pitying tone, if they can give you a ride in their car. Others will assume you don't want to join them in an activity they plan to attend by car. Some people will lecture you about safety; many get defensive, assuming that you are judging them for not bicycling also.

For all these awkward interactions, though, you'll encounter many others who will cheer you on, and some who will be inspired to join you. Just take it all in stride and keep on living your life the way you choose.

The good news, though, is that bicycling is an excellent way to meet people. Joining a group ride, an advocacy organization, or other cyclists who you meet at work or school or on the bike path are ways to make friends with whom it feels normal and comfortable to go out by bicycle to see a movie or take the kids to the park.

Where you live

You'll soon learn the ins and outs of navigating your way around your daily life. Once you've begun bicycling, it will quickly become clear what works well and what you wish were different. Only a few blocks or one major street crossing can make all the difference in whether or not it is easy and fun to ride from your house to the store.

If you work, shop, visit, and play on one side of a busy street without good crossings, and live on the other, you will likely find yourself thinking about ways to avoid this. Perhaps moving is feasible—just as people will move a few blocks so their kids can go to a better school, others choose to move a short distance away so they can more freely choose to ride everywhere they go.

Moving is often not an option; but you might be able to find a new job, school, or grocery store or laundromat that are easier to bike to (this doesn't always mean it is actually closer). Or your bicycle landscape might just be something you learn to live with over time. And advocacy is always an option—sometimes all you have to do is ask (see Chapter 6).

Where your bike lives

"My bike situation dictates my housing situation."
—Austin Horse, Brooklyn, NY

Wherever you live, you'll need to keep your bikes somewhere, and often the type of bicycle you ride will depend in part on your facilities at home. One advantage of a larger suburban property is you are likely to have extra space—maybe even an entire extra garage—for bike storage. Some imported city bicycles are built to withstand being stored out of doors in all weather. If you want to ride a cargo bike and it isn't built to live outside, you'll need to be able to store it on the ground floor, which isn't always possible in an urban apartment.

The simplest way to store your bike is to lean it against the wall. If you live in a very small space—or have nowhere to park your bike at work—a folding bike might be your best bet. Other bike storage solutions for small spaces range from the brilliant to the bizarre. If your bike has a flat top tube, you can make or purchase a sort of shelf to hang on a wall, with two notches to hang the bike on horizontally and a handy space up top to drop your keys and whatever is in your pockets. If your bike is light enough to comfortably lift, you can hang it by the front wheel from a large, rubber coated hook (a few dollars at the hardware store) drilled into a beam in the ceiling. You can also buy a pre-made, expandable tower that clamps between your floor and ceiling, and can hold two bikes, one above the other.

What to wear
Your regular clothes
What you wear to bike should be comfortable and appropriate for what you're doing. If you're biking to the office, wear your office clothes. If you're biking to a class at the gym, wear gym clothes. If you're biking to a party, or to a job interview, or the grocery store, or out on a recreational ride around the country, you should be able to hop on your bike while dressed appropriately for each of these activities.

At the same time, a polyester blend fabric that keeps you suave and wrinkle-free during an air conditioned bus or car commute may turn into a sweaty, stinking prison on a short summer bike ride. The soles of your favorite walking shoes might be too wide to fit easily on your pedals. The seams on any pencil skirt are very much in danger of splitting.

In other cases, you'll likely find neglected items at the back of your closet that turn out to become bicycling staples. A pair of wool slacks and a wool sweater can keep you cozy and repel light rain in the fall and winter; your dress shoes with stiff soles that aren't comfortable to walk far in might just be perfect on the pedals.

Trousers
Trouser legs are in danger of getting caught in your chain. The classic response to this situation is to roll up your right pants leg before you ride. Creative options abound: you might just switch to more narrow-legged pants. Or you might prefer to put a strap around your ankle. Or you could leave your trousers alone and put a chain guard on your bicycle.

Skirts

If a short skirt is more voluminous or flared, it's in danger of flying up in the breeze as you ride. Wearing a pair of shorts underneath your skirt just for the bike trip is one way to avoid showing your underwear; another is to follow the current fashion of wearing leggings underneath your skirt. In the winter, wool stockings provide an excellent layer of warmth.

Skirts that are longer risk getting caught in your spokes or brakes, causing a crash. One way to avoid this hazard is to tie the extra fabric on your skirt in a knot or to reduce the flow of fabric with a large clip. Another is to install a skirt guard over the rear wheel.

On your feet

Shoes with a stiff sole will be the kindest to your feet. Sandals and flip flops are often looked askance at, but so long as you aren't racing around and you're careful not to let them flop off into your gears, you shouldn't have any problems.

High heeled shoes can actually be much easier to bike in than to walk in. The ball of your foot should rests on your pedal in any event, so the heel doesn't come into play until you need to stop, in which case it makes a nice stilt to keep you from having to climb in and out of your seat.

The practice of rolling up the right pant leg, and generally of wearing clothes that are not long enough to encounter your drive train, leads many an urban cyclist to discover the joys of knee socks.

On your head

A cycling cap isn't just a fashion statement, it's functional cycling headwear year-round. The brim keeps sun and rain out of your eyes. A heavyweight one with an earflap will keep you warm in the winter; a lightweight one absorbs sweat and protects your head from the sun in the summer and serves the vital function of keeping your hair from poking straight up through the holes in your helmet.

Layer up

You'll encounter changing temperatures, internally and externally, as you ride, depending on the terrain, the weather, and your effort. Because of this, it's a good idea to dress in layers. In the summer, you may want to be wearing a sleeveless top for riding, but have a shirt or cardigan to put on as you enter an air-conditioned building and your body cools down. In the winter, it's better to have multiple thin layers that you can shed as you ride rather than a heavy coat that will turn into a sauna at the first hill. Arm and leg warmers may look like hipster fashions but are actually quite practical for bicycling, since you can quickly pull them up or push them down as needed. When you ride a bike, you dress less for the weather and more for maximum flexibility to meet the permutations you'll encounter.

Technical clothing

There's a lot of fancy technical clothing out there for riding. If you plan to ride more than 10 or 20 miles in a day, especially if you like to ride hard and fast, by all means get yourself a full on riding kit: padded shorts, a jersey with pockets in the back, lightweight windbreaker, knee and arm warmers, clip-in shoes and moisture wicking socks. If you like the look and feel of technical bicycle gear and if you find it functional for your riding style, there is no reason not to wear it.

But if you'll be mainly riding for daily transportation at a leisurely pace, this type of gear is rarely necessary. There are exceptions, and many technical items, such as rain gear, have their place in an everyday wardrobe, particularly in inclement weather. But there is no need to invest in an expensive new wardrobe in order to ride a bicycle. See what your habits are and choose your purchases wisely.

Padded bike shorts are a popular technical item. Keep in mind that, depending on your body and your bike, padding sometimes pinches and will not necessarily increase your comfort; your first step before resorting to padded shorts should be adjusting your saddle and handlebars. If you plan to put in many hours on the saddle, try shorts with thinner padding first before working your way up to more. If you wear bike shorts, you do not need to wear underwear underneath. Remove them as soon as possible and wash them in between every time you wear them.

Dirt and grease

One of the common clothing pitfalls of bicycling is dirt. There are two main kinds. One is dirt from the road, your tires, and the sooty stuff that wears off of your brake pads. The second is dirt-infused grease from your chain.

Road dirt should come off your clothes handily in the wash. Chain grease is another story. If you have a stubborn chain-ring tattoo on your favorite trousers, soak the mark with a citrus-based solvent, let it seep into the fibers for several hours, and then wash the item as normal.

Chain grease on your clothes can partially be avoided simply by keeping your bike chain clean and well lubed. Dirt from your brakes and tires can likewise be avoided by regularly cleaning your wheel rims with a dry cloth. If it's important to you to keep grease off your hands, keep a pair of rubber gloves with your bike tools and wear them whenever you need to clean or work on your bike.

You're most prone to getting dirt and grease on your hands and clothes while lifting your bicycle, for instance up stairs or onto the rack on the bus. Avoid this by learning to lift your bike gracefully, rather than wrestling with it. One trick is to always stand on the left side of the bicycle while you lift it, away from the drive train. The rest comes with practice.

Riding in all weather

You can ride a bike through most any weather. These tips will help. Listen to your body and your instincts at all times, especially if it is very cold or hot. And it's essential, as with any other form of transportation, to have a backup plan for extremely inclement weather.

Rain

A light rain, particularly in the summer, can be lovely to bike through. Heavy rain storms can also sometimes be fun, though people tend to drive very badly during them.

In cold, wet weather, your main concern should be staying warm rather than staying dry. Any time you wear a raincoat and make any kind of effort on your bicycle, you will end up sweating, and so the trade off between internal and external moisture must be balanced.

If is just drizzling, you may be best off with no raincoat at all. If it is warm out, lightweight synthetic clothing dries quickly, leaving you more comfortable than if you were sweltering in an unseasonable raincoat. If it is cooler out, a thick woven outer layer like a tightly woven coat or a wool sweater is often your best measure; it will shed water and keep you warm even when it is wet.

Real rain, on the other hand, is when technical bike clothing shows its worth. If you own no other piece of technical gear, a bicycle-specific rainjacket is the item to invest in. These are typically made of breathable, waterproof fabric and are equipped with a longer flap in the back, ensuring the small of your back stays dry as you lean over your handlebars. Most have pockets, and many sport zippered ventilation holes in the armpits.

Technical rain pants are another item that many city riders swear by. You can find very cheap, non-breathable ones at military surplus stores, or invest a bit more for breathable fabric and a fascinating array of permutations of zippers and closures. Look for ones that fit comfortably over your regular trousers and that can be taken on and off with relative ease when you are, for instance, standing by the side of the road with a storm approaching quickly.

One of the best and cheapest kinds of outerwear is the rain poncho. One size usually fits all, and attaching thumb loops means the poncho serves as a tent to keep your lower body and feet dry while you ride. If you go this route, you'll really need fenders; rubber boots and/or rain pants are a bonus. The downside of a poncho is quickly discovered in strong winds.

Fenders are essential in wet weather. Water from the sky may get you damp, but the water that your tires throw up from the pavement will cover you with grime. It's possible to buy small, clip-on fenders that will offer some minimal protection, but you'll really be better off with a set of full fenders that wrap partly around your tire and extend nearly to the ground. This is for your own sake as well as the sake of anyone who happens to be riding behind you on a wet day; inadequate fenders will direct a spray of dirty water directly into their face.

Wool socks are especially amazing in the cold and damp, as are any kind of "performance" socks. Neither of these is particularly comfortable when wet, but both are far preferable to cotton in keeping your feet warm.

In wet weather wear shoes with plenty of grip so they don't slip off your pedals. Over your shoes, technical fabric rain booties are nice to keep your feet dry; rubber boots will do as well, though you'll need to prevent water running into them from above.

As for keeping the rain out of your eyes, a visor on your helmet will help marginally; a cycling cap with a brim will help even more. You can also purchase a waterproof helmet cover to keep your whole head somewhat more dry and warm. Some rainy weather riders prefer contact lenses over spattered and fogged glasses.

When it rains it's often darker than normal, and it's a good idea to have lights on your bike at these times as well as to ride extra cautiously.

A note about size: Technical bike gear, including rainwear, is rarely made in women's sizes above 14. You'll find a few things out there, but the options are limited. If you have trouble finding rain gear that fits you, a poncho is one option; or you may prefer to swing the opposite direction and opt for a fashionable wool or waxed burlap coat.

Cold

In cold weather, you have two factors to consider. On the one hand, even if you start out cold, your body will warm up as you ride. But on the other hand, riding will cause the air to rush past you—even when it isn't windy—making you colder, especially your hands, face, and feet.

Most warm winter clothing focuses on keeping your core warm—a giant down jacket, for instance. But your core is what heats up the fastest when you're on a bike. Get too warm, and you'll find your sweat cooling you off too fast when you're going down hills or once you stop.

Unless you are riding in below-freezing temperatures, ditch the parka and layer up. This might entail a lighter jacket over a couple of sweaters, and long underwear underneath all your clothes. You'll also want more, warmer coverage of your extremities, for instance double socks, gloves, scarves, and hats. Military surplus stores are excellent places to get affordable, durable cold weather clothes for bicycling.

A regular scarf can come loose while you ride or produce openings for the wind to get through; try a neck tube or balaclava instead.

When dressing to go out on a cold day, pay extra attention to the gaps between items of clothing that let cold in when you're on the bike: your face, your neck, between your gloves and sleeves, at your ankles, and the stripe on your lower back between your waistband the bottom of your shirt.

Snow and ice
Cycling in ice and snow has its own skill set (and equipment recommendations). People who ride in snowy climates often keep separate bicycles that are set up for winter riding.

For some kinds of snow, knobby mountain bike tires may help you gain traction. But on ice or hard packed snow, smooth tires are better as they provide more surface area to grip the slippery road. In slippery conditions, lowering your tire pressure to its minimum may also help increase the amount of gripping surface on your tires.

Heat
There are two schools of thought about bicycling in very hot weather. One is to wear as little as possible to stay cool; another is to cover up with lightweight fabric to avoid sunburn. Cotton is more comfortable and breathable, and technical lightweight wool has its devotees. Whatever you wear, light colors will absorb less heat, and patterned fabrics will show less sweat.

Drink a lot of water when you're biking in hot weather. Several cups of water before you leave the house will get you started, and then drink more as you ride. Drenching your cap and shirt in water before a ride in the scorching heat can help your body keep cool for longer.

Plan your day to stay cool. Between 6 and 8am is the coolest time of day; peak temperatures are reached between 4 and 6pm, right during the evening commute.

Also, it's counterintuitive, but staying out of the air conditioning will help your body acclimate to the heat. It takes about two weeks to really get used to hot weather, and every blast of AC resets the clock.

Whatever you do, take it slow and easy when it's hot. If you start to feel sick from the sun, stop riding immediately, drink water, and go somewhere cool.. And wear a lot of sunscreen; don't forget that exposed stripe on your lower back.

Taking care of your body

Bicycling doesn't have to be an athletic endeavor, but it is a physical activity. When you begin to bike regularly, you may find you simply need to eat more throughout the day to avoid the dreaded blood sugar crash. Making sure some of those extra calories are from fresh, whole foods will give you more energy and strength for riding. If you sweat a lot, be sure you are consuming enough salt.

Stretch and strengthen

Muscles get tight when you use them. Your body will thank you if you stretch regularly, even if just for a couple of minutes before or after a ride or at the end of your day. Yoga is especially good for staying limber and strong, but the basic stretches you learned in gym class as a kid will serve just as well. Your hamstrings, quads, and hips in particular will thank you for the extra attention.

Bicycling gives you strong legs, but it doesn't do much for your upper body strength or your core. And any form of exercise that builds abdominal strength will help you get up those hills. Improving your overall fitness will make bicycling continually easier and more fun, so go for it.

Finally, riding a bike should never hurt. If you're in pain, something's wrong. You might need to start stretching a particular muscle, tweak the fit of your bike, adjust your saddle, get your cargo off your back, try a new kind of handlebars, or even see a doctor. Regardless, don't just push through the pain; research it and consult an expert.

Crotch health

A few sensational articles have been published over the years claiming that cycling can harm your sexual health. And if you ride for many hundreds of miles each month you are indeed likely to suffer in the crotch department. If you are a more casual rider, however, you will likely only need to worry about your fertility and sensation when and if you actually experience discomfort.

When you first start riding, or when you switch to a new saddle, the bones in your pelvis will be sore for a few days. This is normal; if it is deeply painful, or doesn't fade in a week, adjust your saddle or switch to a different one.

To stay comfortable in the long term, it's important that your seat fit and your bicycle be well adjusted for your body. This is not just a matter of your saddle adjustment; even a centimeter's difference in the angle of your handlebars can affect the comfort of your seat. For more on adjusting your seat, see Chapter 3.

Experiment with different clothes and equipment to make sure you are not over- or under-padding either your bicycle seat or your crotch. Some people can ride happily while wearing anything and on any saddle; others are most comfortable with lots of padding, others with thin padding, others with none at all. Some people find that any clothes with seams in the crotch, particularly jeans, are unbearable. If you experience lasting numbness or pain, see a doctor. You may need to switch to a more upright bike or recumbent.

Also in the crotch department, it's important to be extra attentive to hygiene. This is especially true if you wear synthetic underwear or technical bike shorts, which are ideal bacterial and yeast breeding grounds. Keep your crotch area clean. If you do go for long rides in bike shorts (or ride any distance in warm weather with any synthetic fabric next to your skin), keeping very clean and using a chamois cream (it's pronounced "shammy") can help prevent painful chafing and saddle sores. After a sweaty ride, products like Bag Balm can relieve chapping.

Menstruation

Many women find that menstruation does not affect their bicycling routine in any way. Some enjoy reduced cramps and premenstrual symptoms as a result of bicycling and generally staying physically active. Other women find that their period brings a low ebb in energy and such an increase in physical and mental discomfort such that they prefer taking a break from bicycling for a day or two.

As for dealing with the actual flow, this tends to primarily be a problem for those who have heavy bleeding. Some women avoid using tampons when they bike, finding them uncomfortable and less effective. A popular alternative is the reusable cup. Multiple varieties are on the market, made of either rubber or silicone.

Pads pose a different issue. Thicker disposable pads tend to bunch up uncomfortably. The extra thin kinds work better but suffer wear and tear in the saddle and will need to be changed often. Cloth pads are not usually ideal; they are either too thick, or they shift around while you ride. Some varieties are secured with a snap, but this is not well placed for comfort on a bicycle seat. Some types of thinner cotton pads with an impermeable backing and a non-snap closure exist; they are harder to find but are popular among women who ride.

Mixing it up: Other ways to get around by bike

When you choose to hop on a bicycle, that doesn't mean that bicycling is the only way you'll travel again, ever. Even the most hardcore transportation cyclists mix things up from time to time.

Public Transportation

Public transportation and bicycling can be a winning combination. Transit lines are fixed, meaning they're only convenient if you live near one and then work near the other end of it. A bicycle can help bridge the gap.

In many places, you can bring your bike onto the bus or train, though sometimes this is only allowed during limited hours, or if there is room on board in the designated bicycle spaces.

If bringing your bike on the train or bus is a problem, you have several options. On the cheaper end of the spectrum is getting a beat up but ride-able bike and locking it up out in the elements at your transit stop; some people keep a second beater bike at the other end of the line.

Another option is to invest in a folding bicycle. These bikes fold down small enough to bring with you on public transportation without any trouble, and nearly all transit systems allow them. The best quality ones are quite comfortable and fast to ride and some even have racks so that you don't need to wear your things on your back.

Cars

You might curse the existence of cars while you're trying to share a busy road with them. But most places in North America are built for cars, and doing without one entirely isn't for everyone. By all means, test out all your options, but chances are you have no real choice but to drive some or even most of the time. Many a rural or suburban person who works in a nearby city has discovered they can get their bike commute in and save money on parking by driving part of the way, parking in a lot or a residential street, and riding the rest of the way in to work.

The simplest way to carry your bicycle in a car is in the trunk. Remove the wheels, rest the frame in the trunk or the back seat with the gears facing up, and place the wheels in afterwards. If removing the wheels is difficult or you don't have time, your best bet is to slide the bike in with the back wheel first, drive train facing up, and leave the front wheel and handlebars hanging out the back of the trunk, rotated at more or less 90 degrees. Bring the trunk lid down gently onto the frame (not on the wheel) and use a bungie cord, a rope, or even your shoelaces to secure the lid snugly to the body of the car so it doesn't bounce open and closed while you drive.

If you find you are often driving with your bicycle, it may be worthwhile to purchase a rack. I recommend bicycle racks that attach to the back of your car rather than the top. It is easier to get the bikes on and off, and you can easily remove the rack when you aren't using it. Many different kinds of racks are available, and it is not difficult to find an affordable used rack in good condition. If you leave your bicycles unattended on either kind of rack, be sure to lock them securely, preferably to the rack itself.

Long distance bike travel

Traveling long distances? It can still be done with a bicycle. Bringing a bike on an airplane is cumbersome and expensive. Some airports encourage bicycle connections by providing safe, well-signed routes and even tools for disassembling and boxing up your bike. Others will actively discourage you from riding to the airport.

Most long distance trains and buses allow bicycles; some require you to box your bike and others don't. Triple-check the rules before you go and consider bringing a printout with you; often there are different requirements and fees for different lines and stations, and station staff are not always on the same page. If you have a folding bicycle, your long-distance travel connections on any mode will be greatly eased.

Or you can just skip the connections and ride the whole way. Bicycle touring is enjoying a renaissance in North America, with thousands of people each year pedaling across the country, around the world, or just on weekend trips near their homes. Bike touring is a great way to have an active, affordable vacation, meet the friendliest people, and see the best of every place.

3

Bicycle adoption, care and feeding

For years, I kept only one bicycle at a time. First it was a series of vintage cruisers, then a mountain bike converted to city use, then a fast, custom road bike, and finally that mountain bike again, converted to a longtail cargo bike.

I have loved each of these bikes more than I can say and ridden each of them many hundreds of miles. But there have also been times each of these bikes filled me with frustration and stress. I've been guilty of what I now see as a common mistake: demanding that one single bicycle be and do everything.

The custom road bike was perhaps the most intense example. It was expensive and it was made for me, and I felt some internal pressure to have only positive experiences on it. I loved going fast, but whenever I took it out, I needed to carry a lot of heavy things. The bike was made to fly, not haul, and the heavier the load, the more unbalanced I felt.

It stopped being fun to ride, so I lent it to a friend and got my cargo bike. It was all bliss for a while—I could carry anything at all!—but soon enough the frustration was back. When I was riding with others, I couldn't keep up. A quick trip across town took 15 minutes longer than it felt like it should. The joy of being able to carry anything at all under my own power gave way to the irritation of crawling along even when unencumbered.

So I brought home the fast bike again, took the racks off, and vowed to never again push a bicycle to be something that it wasn't. Now, when I want to carry anything beyond snacks and my wallet, or if I just feel like sitting upright and tootling along slowly, I ride the cargo bike. If I want the thrill of going fast, I put all my errands aside and treat myself to a spin on the road bike.

There are times when one bike is in the shop, and I ride the other for every purpose, and that's liberating in its own way, remembering how far you can push a the limits of what any bicycle can do. But having two bikes works well for me—so well that I'm daydreaming about getting a third, an in-betweener, light and strong enough to carry me over mountains with a sleeping bag and tent on the back. Where to keep it, however, is another question entirely.

Complicated bikes for a simple life.
Bicycling can be as simple or as complicated as you want it to be. Much of that depends on your choice of bike.

If you walk into a bike shop and ask for the simplest bicycle they have, it's likely they'll direct you to the stripped-down, fast steeds with no gears or brakes, much less a rack or fenders. These bikes are fun to ride, but they can end up complicating your life on a daily, practical level, requiring extra creativity and effort to manage even simple tasks like grocery getting and riding in the rain.

If you want to keep things truly easy and change your daily habits and wardrobe as little as possible, consider going for a more complicated bicycle. A bike with some combination of sturdy, step-through frame, built in lights, fenders, a chain guard, a rack, and flat-resistant tires will simplify your transition to bicycling immensely.

For some, simplicity means taking your bicycle to a shop for all routine and special maintenance, and getting components that need as little work as possible. There's something to be said for complexity, too, though, and you may find, as you ride more, that you enjoy the learning and the trial and error of tailoring your bicycle to fit your body and lifestyle; you may even find it more convenient to do yourself. Whichever your preference, this chapter gives you some basic resources to whet your curiosity and get you started.

Choosing a bicycle.

What kind of bike do you need? The short answer is: Any kind. It doesn't matter, so long as you can ride it.

The longer answer is: You need a bike that fits you, that can be kept in good repair, that is suited to your needs and the local terrain and weather, and that feels good and is fun to ride.

Within those parameters, you'll find multiple options, sometimes too many. Keep in mind that there is no single ideal bicycle. Choosing a bike is a matter of figuring out your needs and then finding a bike that will suit them reasonably well.

If you have a search ahead of you, here are some tips for choosing your bike. If you already are happily paired with a bicycle, skip ahead to the maintenance section in the second part of this chapter.

You don't need to marry your bicycle

"Don't try too hard to get the right bike from the start. Tastes change with time, experience and fashion" —Erik Sandblom, Göteborg, Sweden

Don't assume you need to have the ideal bike before you start riding. Waiting for the perfect bike to come along is a great recipe for never beginning to ride at all. When you do find one that fits all your criteria it is likely to be a hefty investment. If this expensive new bicycle turns out to not be a good fit for your body or your lifestyle, you're bound to feel frustration instead of joy when you ride it.

Avoid this fate by shopping around with the goal of honing in on your needs. If you already have a bike that you aren't thrilled with, think about what could make it more fun to ride and make incremental changes one by one with that

Questions to ask yourself

While shopping for a bicycle, think about the following questions. Write down any conclusions that come up and bring the list to the bike shop with you, or keep it next to you as you sift through used bike listings online.

· Do you want to ride fast or slowly?
· How far will you be riding, and how often?
· Are there a lot of hills where you will be riding?
· What kinds of roads will you be riding on—smooth asphalt, rutted streets, or gravel/dirt roads? Will you spend a lot of time on busy streets?
· What do you want the bike to look like? It's okay to care about style and color!
· Will you be carrying stuff on racks on your bike? Will you use a trailer with it? Will you carry children?
· Will you need to carry your bike up and down stairs?
· Where will you park?
· How much do you want to spend?

Even if you do not yet have answers to all of these questions, considering them will better equip you to begin shopping for a bike that meets your needs.

end in mind. If you're totally new to riding, one way to get started is to borrow a bike from a friend or family member who is about your height. Even just renting a bike for an afternoon or test riding a different style of bike at your local bike shop every weekend will help you get a sense of what you like—and, just as important, what you don't like.

Then again, if you know you want to ride, there's something to be said for just jumping into the deep end and getting yourself a bike, any bike. Why wait? Bikes have good resale value, and the bike that frustrates you daily is likely someone else's dream ride. If your shiny new ride doesn't work out, you can sell it and get something else.

You don't have to marry your bike. If your first bike ends up not being right for you, there is no shame in that. Adjust it until it fits your needs as well as it's going to, and then take what you've learned and move on. For most everyday riders, life is a never-ending quest for the perfect bike. There's joy to be found in that, too.

New bikes

New bikes have advantages and disadvantages. They are in one sense easier to shop for, because they are standardized; you will not be faced with a multitude of individual quirks and component choices. A new, low-end hybrid commuter bike from your local bike shop is an easy and affordable entry into the world of cycling, and can be resold for a reasonable sum when you are ready to move on.

Low end bikes are not to be confused with their even cheaper cousins the big box store bikes, which are as a rule not built to withstand regular transportation use. If you are unsure that you want to ride at all, and only want to spend a hundred dollars or so testing the waters, a city bicycle from a big box store might be a good temporary solution. Keep in mind that these bikes do not have any resale value, and there is a danger that your bike may be quite rickety right out of the box. If you do choose this avenue, plan to replace the bike within six months.

Working with a bike shop
You can save money by buying a bike online, but if you'll be riding regularly it's worth spending a little extra in order to develop a relationship with your local bike shop.

That way, when your new bike hurts your wrists or develops a rattle in the first week, you'll have ready help adjusting it to fit and making sure you are happy. You'll always have a place to go with questions, fit help, and repair needs, and when you're ready to buy another bike you'll have the advantage of a guide to the process who is already familiar with your needs.

If there are multiple bike shops in your area, it's a good idea to shop around. You'll want a place you feel comfortable and where they have the things and services you need in your price range. If you have a good interaction with a particular employee, it's fine to ask for them specifically when you go back.

Bike shops can be intimidating to the uninitiated—but they don't have to be. To have a positive experience, there are two rules of thumb:

1. Be prepared. Go in with as clear an idea as possible of what you need, whether this is the exact part and model number or "something has been squeaking since the bike fell over last week." Even if you don't know where to

begin with researching your needs, think them through as thoroughly as you can. Your bicycle dreams will evolve along with your knowledge; for many, it's a lifelong process.

2. Ask questions. If the salesperson or mechanic says something you don't understand, ask them to clarify. If you do happen upon someone who isn't willing to answer your questions, who doesn't listen, or who is trying to push you to buy a racing bike when you are searching for an everyday ride, find another employee to work with or go to a different shop.

3. Test ride, test ride, test ride. Never purchase a bicycle that you have not first taken for a spin and found to be comfortable.

Used bikes

"If you are concerned you may eventually be dissatisfied with new bike, a used bike will be easier to sell for the purchase price."
—Austin Horse, NYC

A well cared-for used bike that has already lasted many miles will likely last many miles more. As with so many manufactured goods, older bikes and parts are better-made than many of their newer counterparts.

Steel frames are heavier, but will last for decades. Aluminum and carbon are less durable and can't be repaired. Before you pay for the used bike you've chosen, run your eyes over every centimeter of the frame. Look for cracks or signs of strain.

Another benefit of a used bike is that vintage bikes are often better-suited for city riding. If three speeds are enough for your purposes, then a vintage bike with a good condition, possibly restored, internally-geared hub, will need less maintenance and result in fewer surprises and breakdowns.

Used bikes, unless you buy them from a shop that restores them lovingly, may need some initial investment beyond the purchase price. If you purchase a bike that has been sitting, lonely, in someone's garage for several years, you will likely need to replace the rubber bits on it—tires and brakes—as well as the shifting and brake cables. You may also find that other parts of the bike, like the chain and gears, are worn out and need replacing. Test the bottom bracket by holding a pedal in each hand and wiggling them to make sure they are sitting tightly in the frame. You may end up spending as much as two or three hundred dollars extra—but this can still be an excellent bargain for a bike that is a joy to ride and will last you for years.

It's also worth noting that you may be able to find yourself a used bike for free or very cheap at a community bike shop. See the maintenance section further down in this chapter.

Types of bicycles
The variety of types of bicycle out there is bewildering. Don't worry about these categories too much; the lines between them can be blurry and defined more by industry marketing than by actual features. What matters is that you have a bike that fits you, that works for you and that you enjoy riding.

City bikes
Just what is a city bike? There is no single answer. In essence it is a bike suited to everyday urban cycling, as opposed to short jaunts on the boardwalk, long, recreational rides in the countryside or racing on tracks or mountain trails.

A classic European-style city bike has full fenders, a rear rack, and perhaps a front basket. It might have a chain guard and perhaps it also has a skirt guard: a casing over the rear wheel that keeps your skirt or coattails out of the spokes.

In North America, bikes adapted for city riding tend to look a little different from this European ideal. They may be sold as a Dutch bike, a cruiser, or a hybrid. They are often road bikes fitted out with handlebars that allow a more upright posture, racks, fenders, wide tires for a more stable ride, and perhaps built-in lights. Almost any bicycle can become a city bike; the permutations and possibilities are endless.

A note on step through bikes
When you think of a bicycle, the image that first comes to mind is likely of a diamond frame road bike, with a straight top tube between the seatpost and the handlebars.

Diamond frames tend to be thought of as men's or boys' bikes. Step through frames, which lack the straight top tube, have become branded in the U.S. as girls' or women's bikes. They were indeed invented for women in the 1800s, meant to accommodate riding in long, heavy skirts and petticoats. Clothing norms have changed, but the association of step through bikes with women and diamond frame bikes with men remains.

There is no reason today for people to choose a frame style based on gender. People who want to ride fast tend to prefer diamond frames, while step through frames (you might also hear some varieties called loop frames or mixtes) are ideal for people of any gender who carry children or cargo on their rear rack, interfering with their ability to swing their leg over. Step-through riders also include people with hip injuries and anyone who simply wants the ease and freedom from wardrobe malfunctions of being able to simply step in front of their handlebars and ride.

Dutch bikes

If you ride short distances, prefer to wear fashionable clothes on your bike, don't have many steep hills to traverse, like to take it slow and smell the roses, and don't want to ever to do any maintenance, then an upright Dutch-style bike with just a few gears may be right for you.

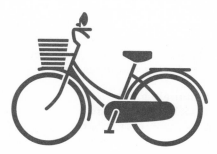

Imported Dutch bicycles are still rare in the U.S. but they are gaining in popularity. They are often but not always step-through frames. They allow you to have a bolt upright riding posture as though you were sitting on a chair or riding a horse. They tend to be heavy, sturdy, and usually do not come with very many gears, since most of them are still imported from the pancake flat Netherlands. They also tend to come equipped with components suitable for city riding including, built in fenders, lights, chain guard, and a dress or coat guard. They are an expensive option in the U.S. but that may change and some cheaper imitators are entering the market.

Road bikes

If you are always on the go, need to hop between commitments all over town, live in a walk-up apartment, aim to replace your gym membership with your daily riding, plan to take your bike camping someday, and need to be able to flip your bike over and fix it on the fly, a light, fast road bike might be for you.

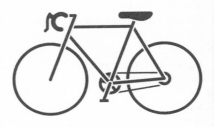

Road bikes are diamond frame bikes, and they typically come with s-curved "drop" handlebars that require you to bend forward to ride. They can be excellent transportation bikes, especially if you prefer to ride fast. When shopping for a road bike, consider that you may want to attach rear fenders and a rear rack. Not all road bikes have the proper attachments that make this process straightforward. Also, many people enjoy the bent-double, aggressive riding posture of a road bike, but it is not practical or comfortable for everyone. If you want a road bike but prefer to sit more upright, consider tilting your handlebars up higher, adding a taller stem, or swapping out your bars, brakes, and shifters entirely.

Mountain bikes

Mountain bikes were at one time a fashionable choice for city riding, and the budget used bike shopper is likely to encounter quite a few of them. If you are less than 5'3" tall, the majority of suitable used bikes you'll find will likely be mountain bikes with 26" wheels.

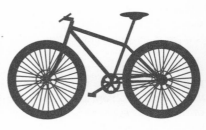

Mountain bikes of the rigid variety can serve well enough as city bikes. They are, however, designed for riding on dirt and gravel roads and trails and single track in the wild, often up and down steep hills. Mountain bikes typically come with knobby tires, which you will likely want to swap out for smoother and narrower ones to improve your speed on city streets. Most mountain bikes come with shocks; you may not want the kind with shocks in both the front and back ("full suspension"). If the shocks are only in the front fork, that can suit for a pothole-ridden commute, but will slow you down; many frames will allow you to swap out the front fork for a stiffer one without shocks.

Mountain bike frame geometry is different from road bikes, and some people find them more comfortable. They generally come with straight-across handlebars rather than the drop bars of road bikes; you'll be more upright than when riding a road bike, but likely still positioned for more speed than a cruiser, Dutch bike, or hybrid. You may run into difficulties attaching racks and fenders to many mountain bikes. Most come with attachment points, but for some you will need to jury rig a way to attach them, which is often not ideal, particularly for fenders.

Touring

A touring bike is similar to a road bike, but heavier and sturdier, and a frame design that makes them more comfortable for long, straight hauls. They tend to be suitably geared for hilly rides, and have the advantages of built-in attachment points for both front and rear racks. They will also take fenders without a struggle, and often have room for extra water bottle cages. All of these features can make them good everyday bikes.

Hybrids

Hybrids are what athletically oriented bike shops tend to keep in stock as "commuters." New hybrids are in the low to medium price range, and they are not necessarily a bad choice for your transportation needs. Hybrids are, as you'd suspect, something in between a road bike and a mountain bike. A hybrid offers mountain-bike style handlebars and brakes, lots of gears, and a semi-upright posture. Some come with a shock-absorbing seat post, which is more gimmicky than useful, but might be nice if the roads you ride on are in bad repair. They can be comfortably ridden for many miles at a time, though they will not carry you as fast as a road bike nor take you comfortably off-road the way a mountain bike can. Hybrid bikes can be very serviceable commuting bikes or bikes for weekend recreation, but once you end up wanting to go faster, ride longer distances, or have more of the trappings of a city bike, it'll be time to move on.

Cruisers

There are two varieties of bicycle called cruisers, though they don't share much in common.

Modern cruisers are essentially beach bikes. They feature wide tires, a single speed, kick brakes (you pedal backwards to stop the bike), a wide, soft seat, and a frame geometry that puts you in a laid back posture. These bikes tend to have snazzy paint jobs and are excellent for a mellow, flat ride down the boardwalk or the bike trail. They generally do not come with racks, but you can easily put a front basket on the handlebars.

Vintage cruisers generally feature step-through frames, an upright sitting posture, three speeds, and heavy steel frames. They are not meant to travel quickly or far, but they are better suited to everyday urban riding than their modern counterparts. These usually do not come with racks, but they are likely to have fenders and a chain guard, and are practically begging to be outfitted with a front basket.

Comfort

So-called comfort bikes are marketed to people who fear that bicycling might not be for them. Unfortunately, this type of bike often successfully convinces them of that. Comfort bikes resemble hybrids, but with an even more upright posture, and swept back handlebars. They come with exaggeratedly wide, cushioned seats, and most are equipped with shock-absorbing seat posts and forks, which increases the amount of effort required to ride. These bikes are not meant to be ridden any great distance or speed or while carrying cargo of any kind.

"Women's" bikes

Occasionally a major bicycle manufacturer will decide to test the market for women bicycle buyers. You can spot these bikes a mile away by their easter egg color paint schemes and floral decals. Their technical design is based on several assumptions about fit, including that women are smaller in stature than men, have narrower shoulders, smaller hands and feet, and have proportionally longer legs and shorter torsos. These assumptions are by no means universally accurate, which is one reason why there are plenty of long-torsoed women and narrow-shouldered men out there riding ill fitting bicycles. Regardless, some shops will steer any female who walks through the door directly to their selection of women-specific bikes. If your dimensions reflect the industry's equations, by all means, take a test ride—no matter what your gender.

Tricycles

People who are seeking extra balance and stability are often drawn to tricycles. But trikes are not necessarily easier to ride than two-wheelers. They are prone to tipping onto two wheels while you turn, and can be more difficult to ride in a straight line on a road with any sideways slope. Nonetheless, some people swear by tricycles, with recumbent trikes—which you can go quite fast on—having particularly fervent devotees.

The trick to keeping your tricycle upright is to lean in the opposite direction as you would on a two-wheeler—away from the direction of your turn, rather than into it.

Recumbents

Recumbent bicycles, or 'bents, are something you either love or hate. On these bikes (or trikes), you sit in a little chair, leaning backwards. Your feet are on pedals in front of you, and your hands control the steering and brakes from your sides.

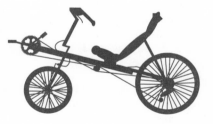

Recumbents are the domain of long distance riders and by the subset of the cycling population who cannot comfortably adjust to regular bike saddles. 'Bent riders are fans of being able to put their foot on the ground without dismounting at stops, as well as the more laid back vantage point these bikes allow. There is quite a bit of fierce debate over the merits of recumbent riding; you're either a recumbent person or you aren't, it seems, and the only way to find out is to give it a try.

Folders

Folding bicycles are beloved by frequent travelers, tiny apartment dwellers, and people who combine bicycling with public transportation. The best folding bikes ride like full-sized bikes and have a small but wide range of gears. Some even have racks and lights built in. A wide range of options are available in terms of sturdiness, ease of folding, ride comfort, and cost.

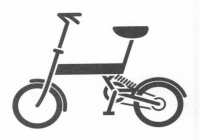

Cargo bikes

"Spend big, expect lots." —Joe Biel, Portland, Oregon

Cargo bikes tend to be heavy, but they can also carry more weight more comfortably. If you need more stuff on a daily basis than can be comfortably hauled on your regular bike, and if speed is not important to you, a cargo bike might be the right choice. All cargo bikes will handle very differently with and without a load, which is worth keeping in mind when you are test riding them. Chapter 5 has a more in-depth section on choosing and using cargo bikes, much of which is applicable even if you are not carrying children.

Longtails

The longtail is the quintessential U.S. cargo bike. Nearly as narrow as a regular bicycle, these bike frames extend several feet longer in the back, with the rear wheel moved back as well. The result is that you can carry larger items than on a regular bike, and keep them centered over the rear wheel in side panniers. The bike's center of gravity is lower, allowing more stability overall.

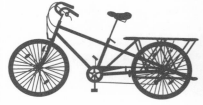

Longtails were invented for the purpose of carrying two hundred pounds of green coffee beans along a mountainous dirt trail in Central America, or to carry sacks of grain down rutted roads in Rwanda. It turns out they work just as well for hauling a set of kitchen chairs, a month's worth of groceries, or two preadolescent children around a hilly U.S. city. They have been embraced as one of the most practical, fast, lightweight, and affordable cargo bike options available.

The variety of longtail options on the market is increasing rapidly. Xtracycle, the original company to introduce them, also makes a kit that can be used to convert your existing bicycle into a longtail. Whatever option you choose, a full-on diamond frame with a straight top tube is not recommended, especially if you'll be carrying anything on the top deck of the longtail that might make it difficult to swing your leg over.

Frontloaders

Frontloader cargo bicycles are a different kind of bike altogether. They are a staple in the bicycle-friendly cities of Northern Europe. Recent years have seen a growing interest in them in the United States, particularly among families. The kind you are most likely to see in the U.S. is the "bakfiets" (pronounced *bock-feets*; the plural is "bakfietsen"), named for its signature wooden box. 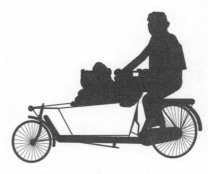 These bikes are stable, but they are heavy. They take some upper body strength to ride, and handle differently than regular bicycles.

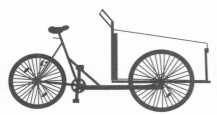

There are other front loaders on the market that are lighter and feel more like riding a regular bike, though their cargo compartments are not as sturdy. Some front-loading cargo tricycles can be found as well, including models that are made in North America.

· When you sit on the saddle and hold the handlebars, with your feet horizontally even with each other on the pedals, your arms should be parallel to the angle of your thighs.

· Your hands should rest about shoulder width apart.

· You must be able to reach your brakes comfortably at all times.

· Your weight should never be on your arms.

· Your seat should be high enough that your foot is flat while your leg is nearly straight. It should not be so high that your legs are overextended or your hips rock side to side when you ride.

· The ball of your foot should rest on the center of the pedal.

· When you're standing over a diamond-frame bike with your feet on the ground, there should be at least a couple of inches between the top tube and your crotch.

Bike fit

As a beginner, you don't need to know too much about bike fit. If you can easily reach both the pedals and the brakes and it doesn't hurt to ride, you're good to go. Have fun!

Most bike shop employees are trained in the basics of fitting and can help you choose a bike that is the right height and length for you. After that, adjusting the saddle position and handlebar tilt are often all that's needed to make your bike work. The trick to adjusting your bike fit is to do one type of adjustment at a time and only make incremental changes. Each centimeter can make a huge difference in the way your bike feels.

Professional bike fitting

If you end up riding many miles at a time, or racing, you may find you want to fine tune the way your bike fits you. There's an art to this, and professional fitters exist who will, for a price, measure your dimensions and abilities with lasers and computers and adjust your bike and its components to fit you, down to the millimeter.

If you are having trouble finding a bicycle that feels comfortable, or if you have a body that the bike industry does not consider "standard," a professional fit is something to consider. A trained fitter will help you learn more about your body, your preferences, and what options are out there.

A note on custom, handmade bicycles
The next step up from a professional bike fit is having a bike made specifically to fit you.

There is a growing industry in the U.S. of custom, handmade bicycles, crafted and fit specifically to your body and needs. These bikes have the advantages of being one of a kind works of art as well as being made and built up with components to your exact specifications. They also have the benefit of being manufactured locally. As a result of these factors, custom bicycles cost thousands of dollars.

An investment in a handmade bicycle will have the best results when you have a very specific and technically detailed idea of what you want from a bike. With custom bikes, you will get exactly what you ask for, and as a beginner you may not yet have the strongest sense of your exact needs. Once you are confident in your ability to choose and adjust an off-the-shelf bike to suit you, you'll be all the more ready to work with a frame builder to create the custom bicycle that will live up to all your wildest, and highly developed, fantasies.

Bikes for all sizes
Sadly, fat prejudice does exist in the bike industry. But there's no need to let this stop you. When bike shopping, it's extra important to find a shop where you feel comfortable and are treated with respect. If you run into problems, bring your business elsewhere.

Many bike shop employees will try to steer bigger-bodied customers towards hybrids. That might be what you want—a slower, slightly more upright ride—but it might not. If you're concerned about a bike being sturdy, look specifically at bikes made for utilitarian city riding, mountain bikes, and touring bikes—they're built to get you up hills and take a beating.

Most bigger-bodied folks won't need a special bike or components. The weakest point on a bicycle is often the rear wheel; if you carry a lot of weight, you may need to eventually get a stronger one.

Bikes for all abilities

Bikes are a flexible medium, and can be adjusted to suit nearly every need. For instance, while on a cross-country bike tour, a friend broke her right wrist. Instead of calling it quits, she had a local shop modify her bicycle so that she could operate both sets of brakes and shifters entirely with her left hand.

A growing array of options exists for "adaptive cycling"—bicycle designs and styles that make human-powered transportation accessible to people with a wide range of disabilities, injuries, and specific needs. The variations out there are as brilliant and creative, as simple and complex as the range of human needs and abilities.

If you have impaired vision, many cities have programs where you can ride on a tandem along with a sighted partner. If you can't pedal with your legs, there are "handcycles"—recumbent trikes that you pedal with one or both arms. A national system of camps uses wide-tired bikes to teach kids with developmental disabilities to ride independently. Limitless variations exist on tandems, tricycles, and four wheelers. Some frame builders are even working on bicycles that can accommodate wheelchairs!

More considerations
Saddles

New riders are often tempted by saddles that are very wide and very soft, like cushy chairs. When you're pedaling, though, these enticing perches are often a recipe for discomfort.

In regards to width, your best option is a saddle that is wide enough to comfortably accommodate both of your sits bones (the two bony protrusions you can feel where your inner thigh meets your crotch). There is considerable variation in this dimension between individuals, and it has nothing to do with your body type—you can have a large fundament and be most comfortable on a narrow saddle, or vice versa. If your saddle is too wide, the sides will chafe your legs when you pedal; if it is too narrow, you'll never find a comfortable seat.

As for softness, the myth is that a cushy, gel-filled saddle will shield your nether parts from chafing. Unfortunately, excess seat padding tends to have the opposite effect, creating more points of contact where painful chafing and saddle sores can occur. Everyone is different, but most people are happiest on either a lightly padded saddle or just hard leather that has been broken in to fit them. Many people prefer saddles with a cut out down the center (available for both men and women), while others find this feature painful. You may need to try different saddles (and different combinations of saddles and trousers and/or technical bike shorts) in order to find what's best for you. Some bike shops allow you to test ride seats—if yours does, take them up on it!

Your seat should be just high enough that your leg is straight when the ball of your foot rests on the pedal at its lowest point, but not so high that your leg locks or that you need to rock your hips back and forth to ride. You'll also want to move the saddle far enough forward that you can reach the brakes without locking your arms. If doing so puts your seat too far forward for comfortable pedaling, then your bike is too long for you.

Saddle angle matters, too. If the saddle nose is irritating your crotch, it might make the most sense, counter-intuitively, to tip it upwards slightly—this pushes your weight further back, onto your butt. If you have the opposite problem, tip the saddle forward a bit—but not so far forward that your weight rests on your arms. If adjusting your saddle tilt doesn't improve matters, then return it to level and adjust your handlebar tilt instead.

Gearing
Shifting gears can be intimidating at first, but quickly becomes second nature. Practice is key. Ride around the block and shift back and forth through your entire range of gears a few times, and you'll get the hang of it.

The gears on your bike amplify the power of your pedaling. If you need to get up a hill or get started with a heavy load, shifting down (that's to a smaller chain ring up front or a larger one in the back) will give you a boost. If you're cruising downhill or on the level and want to go faster, shifting up will transfer more of that power directly into making your wheels spin. Shift just before you begin to go uphill, and the chain will slide more smoothly onto the next gear. You must continue pedaling while you shift.

How many gears do you need? There is a lot of complicated lore and math about bike gearing. It's actually pretty simple. If you live somewhere with hills, or plan to carry anything heavy on your bicycle, you'll be happier with more gears. If you'll be riding relatively flat streets without a lot of stuff, only one gear might be enough, three should be fine, and ten will certainly be adequate.

If you're on the fewer-gears end of the spectrum, you can spend some extra money on an internally geared hub (some vintage cruisers have these as well). These have several benefits: the gearing is protected from the weather and barely needs maintenance. While you cannot shift and pedal at the same time with these hubs, you do not have to remember to shift down before stopping while going uphill.

The electric assist

An electric assist is like having extra gears on your bike. It is fundamentally different from a motorized scooter or moped in that it has no throttle and can't power you up a hill while you sit back and relax. On an e-bike, you're unlikely to top 20mph even when it's maxed out. What it can do is help flatten that steep hill on the way home from the grocery store. If the hills are very steep and what you're carrying is very heavy, that's worth something.

The downside to an electric assist is that the battery is bulky and heavy—meaning that if you run out of juice, or simply don't want to use the assist, you'll find yourself with one more big thing to carry. Regardless, some cargo bike riders are starting to adopt electric assists. Other fans are people who live at the top of a steep hill, or need to avoid exertion for medical reasons, or simply prefer to avoid getting sweaty on the way to work.

If you're curious about electric assists, it's worth taking a few out for test rides. But keep in mind that with enough gears on an unassisted bicycle, you may discover you have all the power you need.

Maintaining your bike

For many new riders, bike maintenance is a black box. But keeping your bike in working order can be as simple or as complex as you want it to be. There is nothing wrong with handing your bike over to a shop every time anything seems a bit off, and this practice is in fact not as expensive as you might think. Likewise, spending a little extra on a bike that rarely needs to be maintained is the best path for many of us. There are benefits to learning a few tricks yourself, though—as you'll discover the first time you discover you have a flat tire after your local shop is closed for the night.

In fact, nothing about bike maintenance is particularly difficult once you have learned how to do it. It doesn't take any special mechanical abilities—just some attention and a willingness to learn, one small step at a time.

You can hand over your bike to your trusty local bike shop and they'll fix what ails it, for a fee. That's a fine option and there is absolutely no shame in never, ever touching your bike with maintenance in mind. There are other ways to go, though, especially for simpler routine maintenance tasks like cleaning your chain and adjusting your brakes, intermediate ones like changing flat tires, and advanced bike wizardry like cleaning and repacking your hubs. I stick to the basics, below, but there are many, many resources for learning everything you want to know about bikes and more.

Community bike projects

There's a different kind of bike shop proliferating in cities and towns around the world. They're called "community bike projects," "bike co-ops," or sometimes funny and whimsical names. You can usually identify them by the smiles and bustling atmosphere inside and the giant heaps of donated bike frames and parts out back.

These are places where anyone can go and get a bike, or bike repairs, or parts, or gear for free or very cheaply. Everything is donated, and most are run entirely by volunteers. There's a catch, though: you'll need to do the work yourself, and you'll often need to trade volunteer hours for parts and frames. Volunteers are on hand to guide you through fixing or building your bike, giving you tips and encouragement step by step as you diagnose your bike repair needs, find the parts, and take things apart and put them back together. It might sound intimidating, but the beauty of bicycling is that nearly everything is easily fixed and there are only a few simple systems to learn about. It's incredibly empowering and a great way to meet people and find out about other rides, events, and activism opportunities.

These bike projects often have a weekly or monthly night just for female and trans identified persons. If your local project doesn't have one, there's no reason you can't start one, even if your bike knowledge is rudimentary. These places are all about people from all different walks of life helping each other make things happen.

Be your own mechanic
If it's more your style to figure things out for yourself in the privacy of your home, why not learn to be your own mechanic? All you need is some elbow grease, patience, time, and a good book or access to the internet, where you can find words, photos, and videos to help you learn to do any bike maintenance task you can dream of.

Here are some extremely basic tips to start you out:

Air up. Tires need the air topped off occasionally; more often in the summer. Buy a floor pump for this purpose or swing by a bike shop occasionally to use theirs. The little portable pumps that you can throw in your bag for emergencies won't get your tires up to full pressure.

Each tire has a recommended range of pounds of pressure—measured in pounds per square inch, or PSI—that's written right on the sidewall. Most tires have a recommended pressure range. Try to keep it within five or ten pounds of the maximum. If you over-inflate your tires, you'll notice you'll start to send chunks of gravel flying. If you under-inflate them, you'll have to work a lot harder to ride, and you risk the dreaded "pinch flat" or snakebite from your tube getting pinched between the tire and the wall of the rim.

Flat tires are the most common maintenance problem you'll have. A time will come when you'll be riding along and hear either a loud pop or a slow hiss, and suddenly you'll have a puncture. Actually, they're a bit of a misnomer. While it's possible for the tire itself—the part that comes into contact with the ground—to wear through or develop a hole in it, most flats are actually caused by punctures in the much thinner rubber tube that sits inside the tire. Most flats are caused either by a piece of glass embedded in your tire that's worked its way through to the tube or else by the tube being pinched between the tire wall and the rim when the air pressure gets too low. Patching or replacing the tube is usually quick and not very expensive if a bike shop does it; it's even cheaper if you learn to do it yourself.

Keep your chain clean. All you need is a rag and a little bottle of chain lube (definitely don't use anything but made-for-the-purpose chain lube unless you're in a real pinch). Flip your bike upside-down, wipe the gunk off your chain and gears, put a drop of lube on each link, and then wipe off all the lube. Voila. If the weather's wet, you might even do this every day. This will keep your gears from wearing out prematurely—they're expensive to replace, so this basic maintenance helps your pocketbook as well as your ability to shift.

Brakes and rims. The more you brake, the more your brake pads wear down. As this happens, they leave a layer of debris on the rims of your wheels. When your rims are dirty, they wear your brake pads down even faster, like sandpaper. It's a good idea to get in the habit of wiping down the rims with a (non-greasy) rag every week or so, and more often in wet weather. Also keep an eye on your brake pads. When they are down to the wear line, have them replaced. If you let them go further, you won't be able to brake easily; and if you let them wear down to the metal, they'll tear up your rims. This is another piece of cost-effective maintenance, as wheels are a lot more expensive to replace than brake pads.

The annual checkup. It's in the nature of screws to come unscrewed, especially as you ride for months over bumpy roads. Brake pads wear down and so do chain rings. Rubber gets old and needs to be replaced. Cables wear out. Hubs need to be adjusted. Derailleurs can get finicky. It's a good idea to bring your bike into a shop for an annual once-over, preferably at either the end of winter or the beginning, or both. Or do an annual checkup yourself, working through the chapters of a bike maintenance book.

Protect your bike

In any city, a good lock is a necessity. Lock your bike up good any time you leave it alone out of doors—on a city street, in your own backyard or garage, or in your house while you're on vacation. Cable locks, however burly, will not do you any good—they can be easily snipped with shears in seconds. Spend a bit more and get a u-lock. These make your bike so difficult to steal that some brands come with insurance.

How you lock your bike matters as well. A bike parking staple or rack is probably your best bet, so long as it's securely bolted to the ground. A street sign is usually safe as well, though if bike theft is rampant in your city, make sure the sign at the top, no matter how high, is wide enough that your lock can't be slid over it, and that the sign is bolted firmly into concrete.

Always lock your bike through the frame and around an immovable object. If your u-lock is big enough, also capture one of your wheels within the lock; wheels are an easy target for thieves. Your front wheel is easier for an opportunist to remove, but rear wheels are more valuable (and expensive to replace). Which wheel you lock is up to you; in very high-theft cities, carry two u-locks so you don't have to choose.

Before your bike ever has a chance to be stolen, write down its serial number. This will be necessary to prove ownership in case it shows up at a pawnshop or is turned in to the police. The serial number is usually etched on the bottom bracket, below where the pedals attach to the bike. Take a photo of yourself and your bike and write the serial number on the back; or email yourself a digital photo and serial number with enough descriptive text that you can easily search for it again.

If your bike is stolen, alert the police. There are also several services on the Internet for registering stolen bikes, and there is a reasonable chance that searching online merchants that sell used bikes might turn up yours. If you don't find it again, your lock manufacturer, homeowner's insurance, or renter's insurance may cover the loss.

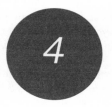

_4_

Carrying things by bike

"Experiment, don't give up, lash it down good, go slow." —Sara S.

When I first started riding a bike, I slung my purse strap across my chest, hopped on, and rode off. I soon graduated to putting the purse in a rickety metal front basket. This was my first bicycle accessory and the most revelatory by far until my discovery, years later, of the rear rack.

My front basket meant speed and freedom. Suddenly I could return my library books on the way to work and pick up a load of groceries afterwards without worrying about marring my professional outfit with a backpack. I could run spontaneous errands and bring leftovers home from a restaurant. In a city built for cars, I suddenly had a taste of how daily life could be not only functional without one, but easier and more flexible.

In the decade since then I've carried a lot of things on my bikes, and done it a lot of different ways. There's no better feeling than arriving across town with your unlikely load intact, be it cupcakes or lumber. I've had my share of misadventures too, and hopefully this chapter will save you from repeating some of them. You learn, over time, to double check that your bungie cords are tight. You also learn that when you apply your brain to the task of carrying something by bicycle, there's very little you can't bring with you.

Wearing your cargo

The simplest way to carry something on your bike is often the same way you would carry it off the bicycle. Put your keys in your pocket, sling your shoulder bag across your chest, tie your sweater around your waist. So long as you keep things close to your body and out of the spokes, you'll often be fine even if you have no other carrying capacity.

You'll find yourself pushing the limits of this method, though, the first time you find yourself trying to ride home with a full grocery bag swinging from your handlebars, banging against the spokes, upsetting your balance, and threatening to send you toppling into the curb.

This scenario tends to lead people quickly to the backpack or messenger bag. Both are easy, noncommittal solutions, requiring no hardware or adjustments to your bike and allowing you to get on and off your bike with minimal hassle. You'll find the bag just as useful when you don't have your bike with you. In fact, you probably already own something like this.

Messenger bags sport a single strap that runs across your chest and over one shoulder. They get their name from their origins among bike messengers who require the convenience of being able to swivel their bag around their body for quick access to the packages inside as they run in and out of an office.

If you don't need easy, constant access to your bag as you ride around, you'll find a backpack to be just as convenient. A backpack is also far kinder to your back and neck, particularly if you often carry heavy items. Whatever you use, you'll be most comfortable with the bag strapped tightly to your body, maybe with a waist strap, and with the weight higher rather than lower.

For bicycling, look for a backpack or bag that is waterproof. If the one you use doesn't keep water out well, stow a plastic trashbag in an easy to access compartment to protect your stuff in case you're caught in a downpour.

Less is often more; and it's a universal truth that the more carrying capacity you have, the more you will find to carry. Sometimes it's nice to travel light, and at these times an excellent way to carry your essentials is a hip pouch. This does not need to resemble the fanny pack of yesteryear if that isn't your style. Several small companies make attractive, waterproof hip pouches specifically with bicycling in mind. Some are made with a slot to handily carry your u-lock while you ride.

Letting the bike do the work

Carrying your belongings on your back has its advantages, but also its downsides. Backpacks make your back sweaty in the summer, and the weight, besides being ergonomically awkward, can lead to injuries.

The good news is that your bicycle can comfortably carry the same load as your back, and then some. Unfortunately, most bikes in North America are still sold without carrying capacity, and adding it is often up to you. Fortunately, there are many options out there.

The front basket

The front basket is iconic, and for a reason.

A basket provides easy access to your things. You won't need to get off your bike or awkwardly rummage through your shoulder bag when you ride up to the drive-through window at the bank or pause to have a snack. You can quickly grab your camera, and no effort is needed to get out your pen to jot down the phone number of the friend you've just run into.

The flimsy woven plastic basket with the plastic flower that graced your bike as a kid might not hold up under the loads you carry today. But a small wicker basket to throw your purse or wallet and keys into is still one of the handiest bike accessories available. Large, sturdy metal baskets are also available, and tend to be quite affordable.

Baskets usually mount to your handlebars. This means that if you ride a road bike with drop bars, the kind that curve forward, a basket might not be your best option, though a handlebar bag might work well. Larger baskets have struts that can be attached to your fork, increasing their load bearing capacity.

A word of caution: if you hit a big enough pothole at a high enough speed, the contents of your front basket will fly up and out, possibly hitting you in the face, possibly breaking all over the road. So if you ride at more than a leisurely pace, some kind of cover is a good idea, or even just a bungie cord or two to keep the contents inside. Also be watchful for any straps dangling through the holes of your basket that might get caught in your front wheel.

More options for the front of the bike
A basket is convenient for small things. But what if you want to carry more weight? While many people prefer to put their weight over their rear wheel, there is a strong faction, including many long distance bike tourers, that prefers to carry their load up front. How you distribute the weight on your bicycle affects how it feels to ride; the choice is a personal one, though some bikes are engineered to be most comfortable carrying the load up front.

The classic way to carry a lot of weight in the front is a front rack that sits low and center over the wheel. The racks consist of bars on which you can hang small panniers. Another option is the porteur rack, a shelf that sits over your front wheel and can serve as the base for a large-ish, boxy bag of the type that is beloved by long-distance cyclists.

Another option is more difficult to find and also more expensive, though quite sturdy. This is the rack or platform that attaches to the bicycle frame itself rather than the handlebars. This type of rack allows you to carry very heavy loads in a way that does not affect your steering. When you turn the handlebars, the rack doesn't move, making for a smoother, more stable ride.

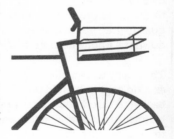

The rear rack
My first rear rack, once I finally got it installed, changed everything for me. I kept a couple of bungie cords strapped to it at all times and used them to hold down whatever I needed to carry: a stack of books, my backpack, a load of groceries, a chair found at the side of the road. This is a strategy that can get you through many years and many quandaries gracefully and happily.

If your bike doesn't already have a rear rack on it, get one. If you have one, use it! You'll be amazed at what it can carry. But use a couple of bungie cords and reasonable caution when you turn, and it also isn't that difficult.

Racks run from very cheap to very spendy. Most bike shops should have at least one basic, $25 model on hand and can attach it to your bike for a small fee. Most racks feature a platform of sorts on top, a bar on each side to hang panniers from, and protrusions near the axle to hook your pannier or bungie cord onto from below. Some racks have holes punched in the back where you can mount a permanent, relatively theft proof, red light.

Installing racks yourself can be a drag. Chances are your bike is not an exact match for the prototype any given rack was designed for. Unless this is the sort of task you love, it can be well worth paying your mechanic to do it for you.

If you carry a lot of weight, you'll need to think about bike maintenance

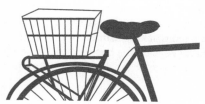 slightly more often than otherwise. Keep an eye on your brake pads—they're working harder and will wear out faster. Also be mindful of your wheels, especially your rear one—if you see any bent or broken spokes, replace them right away, or better yet invest in a stronger wheel.

Bungies and tie-downs

Bungie cords are inexpensive new, but if you don't like them or are really on a budget there are better options. Once you've patched an inner tube more than a few times or suffered a major blowout, it can take on a new, useful life as a tie-down. Some people cut out the valve and tie simple knots or loops. Others leave it intact, wrapping it around their load and rack. Aside from being free—and freely available in bulk at any bike shop—the distinct advantage over a bungie cord is that you don't have a high-stress elastic cord with metal hooks on the end that can seriously injure you.

Whatever you use, strap your cargo down very tightly, with the elastic stretched to its fullest. Believe that whatever you are carrying will use all its wiles to escape, and stay a step ahead of it.

You can use just about anything in a pinch, from your scarf to your sweater to a piece of butcher's twine or ribbon scrounged up by a supermarket employee. Use your shoelaces if you need to. Whatever you use, pull it taut and triple check the stability of your load before you set off.

If you use bungies with metal hooks, don't let them snap back and take out your eyeball. Also, make sure you keep everything out of your spokes, from tie-downs that aren't in use to your long skirt or scarf to your pants leg. Extracting a bungie from your hub is not fun. Being stopped short while in traffic by a hooked spoke can be disastrous, particularly if it is your front wheel that is hooked. Be especially careful to keep all tie downs and straps from dangling anywhere near your wheels.

Rear baskets
My next revelatory upgrade was the $20 folding basket that mounted to one side of the rear rack. The purchase was inspired by an artist friend who had two of these and could regularly be seen trucking around town with her silkscreened tote bag containing wallet and keys in one basket and a grocery bag or stack of letterpress greeting cards in the other. In the rain, she put everything in plastic bags.

As with a front basket, a rear basket is wonderfully convenient. You can just put your backpack, a stack of books, a diaper bag, or a recent purchase in these and ride off. The baskets fold up, which is good if you keep your bike in a narrow hallway. These rear baskets are not extremely durable and are often difficult to mount to your bike. But overall they work great, are a good value, and are about as basic as it gets.

The milk crate
A time-honored carrying technique is a milk crate on your rear rack. These come in various shapes, sizes and colors and can be readily found by the side of the road, behind convenience stores, or holding records in your friend's garage. Attach them to your rack with hose clamps from the hardware store or for a more removable option, strap your crate on tight with bungie cords.

Make Your Own Bike Buckets!

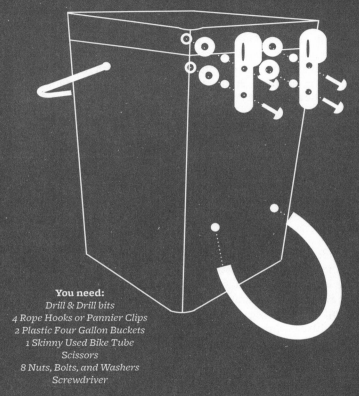

You need:
Drill & Drill bits
4 Rope Hooks or Pannier Clips
2 Plastic Four Gallon Buckets
1 Skinny Used Bike Tube
Scissors
8 Nuts, Bolts, and Washers
Screwdriver

1. Position your bucket so the top sits level with your bike rack without the bottom disturbing your derailleur.
2. Measure, mark, and drill holes (six black holes) so the inner tube will stretch taut when on your bike.
3. Pull the tube through the holes on the bottom and tie knots on each end inside the bucket
4.Bolt your clips or rope hooks in.
5. Attach to your bike rack and test it by riding around the block.

Panniers

Panniers are saddlebags; they're like backpacks for your bicycle, usually detachable, that hang from the side of a front or rear rack.

The iconic city cycling panniers are made by the German company Ortlieb. Their distinctive design is based on rafting bags meant to withstand prolonged submersion. The basic model is just a heavy-duty waterproof bag that rolls down and clips on the top. Plastic clips on the side hook over the top of your rear rack, and a bracket at the bottom keeps the bag from rattling or falling outwards as you turn. They come in bold, bright colors with reflectors on the sides. They're spendy but they last.

Multiple companies now make similar bags, and many have expanded on this basic design with welcome features like external and internal pockets (essential if you ever want to find your house keys or wallet when you need them), and a waterproof hood that stretches over the top of the bag.

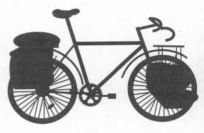

The downside of panniers is that when you get off the bike you must lug them around by their finger-wrenching handle or spine-twisting shoulder strap. This is not a big deal unless you are carrying a lot of weight—a laptop computer, some books, a double load of groceries. If you spend a lot of time walking with all your things in between getting on and off the bike, you may be happier with a backpack and basket combination.

You might also run across touring panniers. These are not always waterproof, and have a great number of internal and external pockets. They feature rugged hardware and—of course—nowhere to clip a shoulder strap.

Sometimes people will use a cable lock to keep their panniers attached to their bike; they just have their stuff in another, more walking-friendly bag inside the pannier. This is a good option if you live in a place where you don't worry about the cable or strap being cut and the pannier disappearing.

Transverse panniers—a staple Dutch bicycle accessory that permanently attaches to your rack—are great for this. You can also purchase square pannier-baskets that are shaped to fit a single grocery bag and intended to be left on the bicycle in low-theft areas.

A somewhat dizzying array of panniers is now becoming available that more closely resemble fashionable purses and briefcases, or conversely that are made of oilcloth and suitable for rugged outdoor use. These are all very different in their attachments and closures as well as their aesthetics. When choosing a pannier for daily use, a primary consideration should be how easily it can be easily opened, closed, and taken on and off the bike multiple times a day.

A note about kickstands

Aside from a rack, the one investment that will instantly improve the way your bike works for you is the kickstand. For under ten dollars and less than five minutes spent fiddling with a wrench, the kickstand will change your life. No more returning to the sign you've locked your bike to only to find it lying helpless on the ground. No more awkwardly holding your bike one-handed while struggling into your rain pants mid-commute.

There are two kinds of kickstands: the most common one mounts onto your bottom bracket—the part of your frame that's between your pedals. This is fine for light use—picking up a few groceries, or taking your laptop to work or your books to school.

A sturdier option is the load-bearing kickstand that mounts to the rear triangle on the left side of your bike. This will keep your bike upright even though you've just balanced a box full of books from the library sale on your rear rack.

Yet burlier is the double kickstand. It costs more but will further revolutionize your life. This kickstand sits at your bottom bracket; when engaged it lifts your rear wheel off the ground and creates a tripod between its two prongs and your front wheel. This is an essential investment for cargo bikes and anyone carrying children. It's also handy for fixing flats on the fly. Triple kickstands exist as well.

Trailers

If putting racks on your bike is proving troublesome, or if you want to have the option to carry bulkier items than your racks can handle, a trailer is an excellent option.

Trailers are easy. You hitch them on, load them down, and ride off, feeling stable and only slightly more encumbered than before. When you're pulling the trailer, slow down on turns. Take it easy on hills. And remember that you're longer than you used to be.

Kid trailers

Trailers built for carrying children have a distinctive upright shape, cloth seats and basic seatbelts inside, and an aluminum frame with a roll bar surrounded by a cloth cover; some have a clear plastic "window" at the top that rolls up to let air in through a mesh screen. For carrying actual kids (or your dog), see Chapter 5.

For carrying cargo, a used kids trailer is usually a good, cheap bet, with little to no modification needed. They have the added benefit of inspiring anyone driving past you to give you a bit of extra room.

These trailers are abundant, gathering dust in garages all across the country as their original passengers outgrow them. In most places you should be able to find a used model for $25 to $100, depending on its condition and demand, at a yard sale or online. Look for one with wheels that don't wobble, screws that can be tightened, inflatable tires, and exterior fabric that's in good enough condition to keep the elements off your stuff. In order for the trailer to be useful, the hitch needs to be in working order.

Modification possibilities are endless. You can maximize your capacity by removing the seat. Some people remove the fabric and make a new bottom out of a sheet of plywood cut to fit. A giant plastic tub can keep your belongings out of the elements.

Cargo trailers

There's a blossoming of cargo trailers on the market, new and used, high end and low. You'll pay $300 to $600 for most new ones; it's possible to

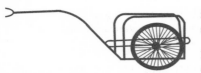

find cheaper ones, but you'll sacrifice sturdiness and durability.

For light, everyday uses, like weekend camping trips or stocking up on bulk flour and peanut butter, a lightweight, fabric-sided trailer should be fine. But be cautious when shopping: some lower end (though not necessarily cheaper ones) are held together with plastic parts, reducing their weight limit significantly.

If you'll be carrying heavier things, even occasionally—furniture shopping, helping out on bike moves, cleaning out your garage or bookshelves, bulk grocery shopping for the neighborhood, carrying an adult sitting on a stool playing the banjo, or the hundreds of occasions that come up over the course of a year that might otherwise send you straight to your local car-sharing service's sign up page—get something a little sturdier.

A workhorse trailer will have a wood or metal floor, and should have all metal attachments. Some kinds come with full sized bicycle wheels; others feature metal guards above the wheels for more easily carrying wide loads. Other trailers are long and trussed like a bridge, able to carry hundreds of pounds. Most trailers have two wheels, but a few have a single wheel. These are small, light weight and don't take up much storage space. Not everyone likes the way they feel to ride with, and you must use caution and slow down when turning.

The trailer hitch
Before choosing a trailer, make sure it has a hitch that plays well with your bicycle.

On many cheaper trailers, the hitch is a hard plastic clamp that attaches to the rear left triangle of your bike frame or seatpost. This is easy to put on and remove, but does not hold up well under very heavy loads; also, some bicycles have design elements that are not compatible, and some racks and kickstands may also prevent you from using this hitch.

Sturdier, though less convenient, is the hitch that is attached to your rear hub. You can remove and attach the trailer easily, but must remove the wheel to move the hitch to another bicycle. This type of hitch places quite a bit of strain on your wheel; keep an eye out for bent or broken spokes as a sign you need to upgrade to a stronger wheel.

Some hitches attach to your bicycle's seat post, and are very functional unless you have a particularly short bicycle or if it interferes with carrying items on your rear rack. A seat post hitch is good for heavy loads, but make sure your trailer is loaded evenly side-to-side and front to back as it will pull on your bike. Balance is everything.

Guerilla cargo tactics
Heavy things
Whenever you're carrying an unusually heavy load, it will feel wobbly at first, and you may wonder how you will manage it. Your body will learn the trick of stabilizing it quickly, though—it tends to take five or ten minutes to adjust. The faster you go, the smoother your ride will feel. Stopping and starting again will be the most difficult part, so if you need to carry something difficult, plan your route accordingly.

The best way to carry weight is low and centered over the wheel. If your weight is too far back or forward it will make your bike squirrely to handle. Some swear that heavier loads are easier to carry up front.

If a lot of your bicycling involves carrying heavy stuff, seriously look into investing in a cargo bike or tricycle. See Chapter 3 for a rundown of your options.

Fragile things
"It's impossible to not jostle something when it's strapped down, no matter how careful you are. I've carried many fancy cupcakes on bikes, both successfully and unsuccessfully. The successful times, I've had a canvas tote bag with a flat bottom that is big enough for the cupcakes container to sit level. You'll need to hold the bag or hang it from your handlebars so it can swing lightly. Swinging lightly is key, strapping down is what causes problems." —Miriam R.

Remember the exercise you did in grade school where you packaged up an egg and dropped it off the school roof? You'll have a similar challenge next time you buy eggs at the grocery store. Or when you offer to bake a cake for a friend's birthday. Or when you take a leisurely summer cruise out to your favorite berry patch and then want to get your seven pounds of blueberries home in berry rather than juice form. Or when you try to bring home a bouquet of flowers for your sweetie.

One peril met by fragile items is simply getting jostled around in your bag when you ride over potholes or tilt to turn a corner. Eggs and light bulbs will survive just fine so long as they are put away compactly, so that they aren't free to rattle around and knock into other stuff. Soft fruit like bananas, on the other hand, should be packed no less snugly but should be surrounded by something that won't bruise it, like a bag of lettuce or a sweater.

The other danger fragile items face is road vibration. In the case of berries or flowers, your body is often going to be the best shock absorber; carry these in a backpack rather than a pannier.

Anything that can't be stabilized on all its surfaces, like a cake, will be better off firmly stuck to a plate that's in a plate-sized box that's cushioned with a blanket and sitting in your trailer or on your rack as you ride extremely slowly and carefully over the shortest distance possible. You can eke out a little extra shock absorption by letting some air out of your tires.

Your beverage

It's always nice to have water around when you ride, and when you are going any distance and speed in hot weather, water becomes essential.

Many bikes come with a water bottle cage, or mounts to attach one. These are cheap to buy and easy to install. They are designed to hold the type of soft plastic water bottles you can buy at bike shops. Some water bottle cages—the bulky plastic ones—can hold a metal water bottle, though these have a tendency to pop out and roll across the road at inopportune moments. You might be better off with your hard plastic, metal, or glass beverage container in a pannier, perhaps one that's partly unzipped where the bottle can easily be reached at stop lights.

If you like to carry your coffee or tea with you while you ride, it's possible to purchase a bicycle-specific cup holder that attaches to your handlebars and holds a tapered cup conveniently close at hand. With a little ingenuity, you could also make your own.

Carrying other bicycles

The time-honored method for carrying a second bicycle is ghost riding. While riding one bicycle, you carefully guide the other bike along by grasping its stem (that's the part that attaches the handlebars to the frame). This requires some mojo and upper body strength. It's best to keep the second bike to your left so that your right hand is by your own rear brake; that way if you have to stop suddenly you won't fly over the handlebars.

If you have an Xtracycle, you're in luck—its panniers were designed with this need in mind. Strap the front wheel of the bike you're towing into the pannier (tightly!); the rear wheel rolls behind you.

Instructions abound on the Internet for making a DIY tow hitch for the rear rack of any bicycle. You remove the front wheel of the bike to be towed, drop the slots on the fork onto the hitch, strap the wheel to your pannier or back, and ride off.

If you have a trailer or cargo bike, you have two options. One is to take the wheels off the second bike and lash it down as well as you can. If bicycles were people, they'd be all elbows and knees, and it can take some finagling to keep the drive train away from your trailer wheel and prevent a rogue handlebar from scraping the ground. If you have the space, it's easiest to stand the bicycle upright on its two wheels, as though it were about to ride off, and lash it down tightly in that position.

How to move by bike

To the uninitiated, moving house by bicycle sounds crazy. Those who have participated in a bike move know the truth—it's faster, easier, cheaper, and more fun than moving with a rented truck and a couple of strong friends.

A bike move is a social event. It's a barn raising, a housewarming party, and a parade all wrapped into one. Numbers are what make it work. When you have 15 friends carrying your belongings out to their bikes, strapping down their loads, and then bringing everything inside at the destination, a move suddenly becomes efficient. It may take a bit longer to ride to your destination, but you save a huge amount of time and energy when you don't have to make twenty trips on each end to carry all your boxes to and from a truck.

The best way to learn the ways of the bike move is to participate in someone else's. If you're a pioneer, here are some tips to get you started:

1. Set a date and invite people. Do this at least a couple of weeks in advance, and remind people again a day or two before the move. If you're comfortable with friendly strangers helping out, promote it widely in your local bicycling scene. Plan it like it's a party. And it really is a party on wheels—you may have to make this clear in the invitation.

2. Have all your packing done by the day of the move. Loading everything up should take about an hour. Be sure to label anything that shouldn't be moved.

3. Food is key. Provide coffee and donuts at the beginning of the move, and beer and pizza at the end.

4. Plan your route in advance to avoid steep hills and high-traffic streets as much as possible. Try to ride the route the day before your move to make sure there are no construction detours.

5. Have extra bungie cords and tie-downs on hand for people to use. If there's a chance of rain, provide tarps.

6. Plan for the big items. Take an inventory of large items like beds and refrigerators and try to make sure enough friends with large bike trailers are able to be on hand. It's cool if you need to borrow someone's truck to finish the job, but don't underestimate the ingenuity of your movers.

7. Take pictures and share them online! The more people move by bike, the more people will want to move by bike...

5

Family bicycling

"Biking is easy. Having kids is hard!"
—Emily Finch, Portland, Oregon, car-free mother of 6

My personal experience with family bicycling is nonexistent. But the family bicycle movement is spreading like wildfire, and when I put out a call for advice the response was overwhelming. Much of this chapter consists of the words of these pioneering, enthusiastic bicycling parents.

These folks represent a wide range of experiences, from being the lone cyclists in a rural area to navigating the streets of the bike friendly cities of the Pacific Northwest. Many of them own cars, some only bike recreationally, and others are resolutely car-light or car-free. Some of their advice is complementary, other times they contradict each other. Your own experience will no doubt vary—and there is no right or wrong way to do any of this.

The family bicycling revolution
"We began riding in the summer of 2011 as we transitioned to a car-lite lifestyle. We were hoping to save money on our automobile expenses and live a more community oriented life."
—Stacy Bisker, Huntington, West Virginia (kids aged 9, 8, 5, and 2)

"We ride to spend time together, to take in the sights, smell the ocean, smile at other riders and walkers on the trail. We ride for small adventures to the beach or on the greenbelt trails through the city. We ride for donuts. We ride to piano lessons because it's faster than driving, more scenic, and makes our cheeks rosy." —Kevin Turinsky, Anchorage, Alaska (kid aged 12.5)

"Taking the bike is fun! We're all happy and relaxed and talking with the kids doesn't distract me on the bike the way it does in the car. I'm also very motivated by avoiding car traffic and not having to look for and pay for parking. It's also a great form of exercise—and my only form of exercise these days." —Madeleine Carlson, Seattle, Washington (kids aged 4 and 2)

"We try to let our older kids be more free roaming like we were in the 70s. That is definitely not the norm these days for other parents but we usually get kudos, if anything, for that stance. The kids—especially the older ones— almost always prefer to bike."
—Dan and Kirsten Kaufman, Portland, Oregon (kids aged 12, 9, and 4)

"Biking is an integral part of our lifestyle, it's faster and more efficient than walking, offers more convenience than relying on bus schedules for most trips and does a great job of keeping us active and in shape. It is easy to sit on the sidelines and bemoan the politics of oil and the injustices of war. I feel that being car-free I am accountable to my children for their future."
—Sarah Noga, Arlington, Washington (kids ages 12, 5, and 1)

For many of us, riding a bike is sweetly nostalgic of our first taste of freedom and independence. But in recent generations, busy roads and an increasingly indoor, online culture limit kids' range of motion even in their own neighborhoods. In 1969, 48% of five to 14 year olds walked or biked to school. By 2009 this number was 13%.

Nowadays, when kids come along, even the most resolutely car-free tend to get cars. And it's no wonder. When a baby is born, suddenly at least one parent can't go anywhere without both the kid and a large bag full of diapers, toys, changes of clothes. As kids get older, someone needs to bring them to daycare, school, camp, soccer practice, birthday parties all over town. Family bicycles are not yet commonplace in North America, and our streetscapes are often anything but kid friendly.

In the face of this adversity, there's a burgeoning family bicycle movement. Many of these bicycling parents are determined that their kids grow up with the values, health, and independence that bikes can afford. Other parents are motivated to rediscover their own childhood joy of bicycling, seek a slower paced life, and find a more satisfying, economical, and healthy seat for their daily rounds than the one behind a wheel of a minivan.

Getting started

"We are new to bicycling and new to family cycling. It was at least 10 years ago I was last on a bicycle. We began the process with a lot of thinking, talking, reading, and eventually just trying." —Stacy Bisker, West Virginia

"The hardest part about starting was getting over the assumption that it's not possible. [It was always] too far, too steep, too many cars to bike to places we've previously visited by car." —Madeleine Carlson, Seattle, Washington

"The hardest part for me was just good old fashioned fear. The family member well-meaning "what-if" questions kept me up at night. What if the baby gets sick? What if it's snowing? What-if... What about... Well none of that is real. It's just like anything else. If a what-if comes up, we deal with it. The car was no magic-measure of security. If worst case something comes up that makes it impractical to bike or take transit to we can rent a car for a day. Like I said, no big deal." —Sarah Noga, Arlington, Washington

Getting started bicycling with kids, like bicycling on your own, comes with a learning curve—and with an added layer of social and logistical hurdles.

But many parents find that the greatest leap is simply deciding to begin. Once they start it quickly becomes hard to remember the obstacles that had seemed insurmountable. In their place, new and unexpected challenges arise, of course. But despite my best efforts to find these out, most parents interviewed for this chapter dwelt far more on the things that became easier and more fun after they began bicycling with their families. I was surprised to hear few complaints about dealing with weather, tantrums, family disapproval, and busy schedules. In fact, several parents expressed that reliance on the bicycle simplified their social life rather than complicating it.

Baby on board
Pregnancy

Many women continue to ride a bicycle throughout their pregnancy; one parent who contributed to this chapter rode her bicycle to the birthing center while in labor, weathering four contractions along her 20 minute ride. The new family came home in a pedicab.

If you have the medical go-ahead to stay physically active during your pregnancy, there is no reason not to continue cycling. Regular physical activity that is built into your day, like bicycling, can help you to handle the physical discomforts that often come with pregnancy, from nausea to swollen feet to mood swings. Cycling can also help you to keep your energy up and maintain your fitness in preparation for birth and what comes after.

As your belly grows, make room for it by switching to a bicycle that allows you a more upright posture, like a cruiser or a Dutch bicycle, or by raising the handlebars on your regular bike. A more upright posture will also help keep you feeling stable as your balance shifts. You may want to add gears as well.

Incidentally, the bicycle types that are most comfortable to ride while pregnant are often the ones best suited to carrying children. Shop for family bikes now, before the baby arrives, while you still have the time and energy. As your pregnancy progresses you'll likely find yourself riding more slowly and avoiding lifting your bike; plan to adjust your routine accordingly. This, too, is good preparation for the pace of life with a baby.

During and after your pregnancy, it's important to listen to your body—and your medical team—when it comes to how much time, if any, you spend on a bicycle.

Riding with your infant

Many parents start riding with their infant right away. Others wait a few months or a year. Before your child can hold their head up, they can be carried in a carseat, either in the bicycle trailer behind you, or in front of you in the bed of a front loader cargo bike. Your car seat carrying solution will depend on what kind of bicycle you plan to ride with your child as they grow.

Bicycle helmets are, in many states, legally required for all children, whenever they are being carried by bicycle. However, they are not manufactured for children under a year old. And it is actually unsafe to put a helmet on a child whose skull is still developing, who is resting in a carseat, or on or any kid who can't hold their head up. As with everything related to carrying kids, it is up to you and your team of experts to decide what is best for your family.

Carrying your child on your bicycle
Once your child is able to hold themselves sitting upright for extended periods, they can be carried in a bike seat.

Want to convert your own bike into a kid carrier by putting a seat on it? There are two basic kinds of child seat: front and rear seats. Many parents of multiple young children have both.

Front seats
"I highly recommend using a front carrier, where the child sits on a seat that is attached to the top tube, and has a foot rest for them. They are nestled in between your arms so they can't fall off. This allows you talk to them, and gives them a great vantage point to watch everything you are seeing. It allows you to discuss bike riding rules and tips with them in "real time." You can easily talk with them rather than shout over your shoulder like a bike trailer forces you to do." —Kristi Wood, Anchorage, Alaska (child is age 6)

"I love front seats—it's wonderful to have a small kid right in front. The only change I had to make to my bike to accommodate the seat was a longer stem when my son's knees got too cramped." —Madeleine Carlson, Seattle

Increasingly common, especially for smaller children, are seats that mount on the front of the bike so that a small child can sit between you and the handlebars. These are loved by many parents for the sense of both protection and conversation they afford. They are loved by children for the sheer joy of being at the front of the bike with the world rushing past. (Windscreens can be purchased for some models for rainy or cold days.)

When choosing a front seat, consider how you will mount it to your bike. This depends both on the type of seat and the type of bicycle you plan to use. The basic distinction is that some of these seats mount to your frame—resting on the top tube—while others mount to your steering. The steering-mounted ones can make the bike somewhat more difficult to control, requiring more strength, but some bike frames make them necessary.

Rear seats

The most widely available seats mount on the rear rack, and can hold kids from a young age up to 75 pounds. These seats come in a lot of varieties; some offer quite a bit of support and may be better for kids that are less good at sitting up on their own. Once you've graduated to a rear seat, you can still easily chat with your kid. If you want to keep an eye on them, a handlebar mirror will help.

There are many different kinds of these available. They are typically mounted to your rear rack. You can also mount them to the deck of a longtail cargo bike, though models built for this are limited and most require some fidgeting. Rear seats are more conventional than front seats as well as easier to find. Your child will eventually grow too large for a front seat, at which point a rear seat may be your best option if they are not yet ready to pedal along with you on a tag-along bike. If you decide to go for a rear seat, consider converting your bike to a longtail (see below). This will improve your overall carrying capacity and give everyone a bit more space.

There are some down sides to rear seats as well. In some cases, a rear seat will interfere with your ability to hang panniers from your rack; others place your child so close to your seat that you will not be able to wear a backpack. Some people find they make the bike top-heavy or hard to balance while getting on and off. And a real downside is that with a child (or even just the seat) on the back of your diamond frame bike, it can be difficult just to get on and off the bicycle.

Getting on and off the bike

If you ride a diamond frame bike (with a top tube that runs straight between your seat and handlebars), you likely get on and off the bike by swinging your leg over the back tire. Mounting a child's seat on the back of the bike will have the immediate effect of making this simple act immeasurably more difficult. Without too much weight on the bike, you can tip it sideways to lower the bar, but when you have a 30 pound kid on the back this also becomes less of an option.

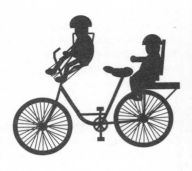

This is where the brilliance of the step through frame becomes most apparent. These are highly recommended for anyone who regularly carries kids or cargo on the back of their bicycle.

If you don't have a step through frame, getting on and off the bike while the kid is on the back may always be awkward. But it can be done.

If your kid is old enough and doesn't need to be strapped in—for instance, if they are sitting on the deck of your longtail—get on the bike first and hold it steady while they climb on.

But most likely, you'll find yourself loading your kid into the child seat and then doing a kind of balancing gymnastics maneuver to thread your leg up and sideways over the top tube while holding the now heavily-loaded bike steady with your arms. Several parents assured me that regular yoga practice really does make this easier.

One way to make getting on the bike easier is to start by standing on a curb while the bike is on the street. A curb may also help with the dismount. Eric Moody of Portland advised, "hold the handle bars and saddle while straddling the bike and then, with great flexibility, pull one knee up and over."

Equipment-wise, just as with any cargo bike, a good, solid kickstand will help a lot with loading and unloading your squirmy cargo, especially if you can kick and un-kick the stand from astride your bike. For even more stability, get a two or three prong model. See Chapter 4 for a more in-depth discussion of these wonderful devices.

Trailers

"When the toddler has fallen asleep, the trailer is a ready made nap bed. I always brought a book in my backpack because it happened quite often. I would get some good reading in and my son would get his afternoon nap."
—Travis Wittwer, Portland, Oregon

If you plan to carry your child or children in a trailer, consider purchasing one made specifically for the purpose. These come in narrower models that hold one child, and wider ones that hold two. They feature a canvas seat with a five-point harness (or two) to strap the kids into the bike. Another feature is a rain/sun cover over a high crossbar that provides room for the kid to sit upright. Some trailers are designed to double as strollers, with a removable push bar and third wheel at the front.

All children-specific trailers have two wheels, which makes them stable and extremely difficult to tip over, though speeding down a steep, curvy hill is never recommended with any kind of trailer in tow.

One of the downsides of trailers is they are bulky and not as easy as an unencumbered bicycle to store in say, a cramped garage or bring through the door of a house. Hitching and unhitching a trailer, if you don't bring it with you everywhere, is an extra step that some find annoying on a daily basis. If you live in an area where theft is a concern, trailers are also not always easy to lock up.

See Chapter 4 for more about what to look for in trailers.

Cargo bikes

A cargo bike combines the best of both worlds. Kids have a bit more room in a trailer, and you can still keep them close, on your own bike, while still being able to carry other kids of cargo, whether it be a diaper bag or groceries.

The basic cargo bike options are described in Chapter 3. Many more varieties exist; most are wonderful, but not every type is for every person. If you're in the market for one of these bikes, be sure to peruse the section below on cargo bike shopping tips.

Longtails

"We're in the process of outgrowing the city bike so a month ago I got a Surly Big Dummy and love it! It's a lot of bike, but it has a lot of gears. So far the thing I love most is being able to haul two kids and their two balance bikes easily around. Previously, I had to hook up the trailer and shove the balance bikes in there, and I have to admit I hate dragging the trailer around."
—Madeleine Carlson, Seattle

"Our typical full family ride uses four bicycles. The two eldest children ride independently, the two youngest ride on our Yuba Mundo with an iBert front seat, PeanutShell rear seat, on the deck, in the trailer, or a combination of any of these. My husband rides his own mountain bike. When I ride with our four children without another adult the same set up may apply, but recently I have preferred to fit them all on the Yuba Mundo in specific situations. Sometimes the children are exhausted and need to be passengers. Other times the roadways, weather or darkness factors may make riding together a safer option. This is working ok for us right now. It's physically possible thanks to months of riding and gradually adding weight and experimenting with setups." —Stacy Bisker, West Virginia

Longtail bicycles are quickly becoming the classic kid-hauling cargo bikes, proving a sturdy alternative to a minivan. You can read more about them in Chapter 3; in short, though, a longtail is like a regular bicycle with a frame extension that places the rear wheel several feet farther back and gives the bicycle a lower center of gravity. Most varieties sport a wide deck atop the rear wheelbase, upon which kids can sit, and two large panniers or ledges for carrying hefty items below and alongside the deck.

Longtails are one of the more affordable family bike options. They can be stored in a relatively narrow space and carried up and down stairs if needed. They also ride similarly to regular bikes, though some parents find them difficult to balance when carrying the bulk of the weight above the top deck, as when children are astride.

There are many ways to carry a kid on a longtail. For young children, you can still mount a front seat between you and the handlebars. One or even two rear seats can be mounted to the top deck. The mounting hardware for most rear seats is not compatible with longtails, so some creativity is required to mount the seat securely.

Older children can sit directly on the top deck. They will be most comfortable sitting on a cushion (waterproof ones are designed just for this purpose). It's also a good idea to install footrests and to mount a set of handlebars below your seat for your passenger to hang onto while you ride. A sturdy double kickstand is essential.

If your longtail has a step-through frame, it will make getting on and off much easier. In addition, a bike that affords an upright riding posture will improve your ability to balance the bike comfortably with top-heavy loads.

The best longtails are the Xtracycle and the Yuba Mundo. Yuba makes sturdy, one-piece longtails that can carry many hundreds of pounds. Xtracycle makes a variety of bikes, all longtails, in multiple sizes and for multiple needs. They also make a kit that you can use to convert the bike you already ride into a longtail.

A variation on the longtail is the Madsen bucket bike. This is basically a longtail frame with a large plastic bucket that sits low over the back of the bike and which has seats for as many as four small children. In the bucket, the kids have room to play and can face each other; and being able to carry the weight of the children and cargo lower to the ground improves stability.

Frontloaders

Just as many parents prefer children's seats on the front of their bike rather than the back, many prefer to carry their kids ahead of them in a frontloading cargo bike rather than behind them on a longtail or in a trailer. This positioning facilitates conversation as well as keeping an eye on what your kid is up to and may give you a better shot at preventing them from removing their helmets and throwing their books overboard. Nearly all of the models described below either come with or have available a variety of options for cargo container, locking compartments, seating and straps, and rain/sun covers.

The handling on front-loading bikes often takes some getting used to; the longer the bike the greater the difference with what you are used to. Some parents report that keeping a fully loaded bakfiets upright requires lots of arm strength and feels extremely wobbly and difficult to pedal at first. They quickly become used to the way bakfiets ride, they say, even if it takes a while longer to build the strength to pedal it everywhere. The trick is to steer the bakfiets like a car, rather than leaning it like a bike.

There are several options on the market for front-loading bikes and trikes; most are imported and quite expensive, though these also tend to be the sturdiest and best-designed.

The most well known front loader in the U.S. is the Dutch bakfiets, with its signature wooden box (Note: bakfiets is pronounced "bock-feets" and is the singular form of the noun in Dutch—the plural is bakfietsen.) The term literally means "box bike" and is a generic category, but there is also a company by the same name that makes a popular model. Imported bakfietsen have some major advantages: Huge cargo capacity (you can easily carry a reclining adult, or two or more children plus a week of groceries in the box). They are well made, with high-quality, enclosed components, which means that maintenance is rarely needed and you can park them outside in the rain year-round without rust taking over. And they're sturdy, built like tanks.

The major downside to bakfietsen is that they are heavy—as much as 100 pounds empty. They were created for trundling kids and cargo around the pancake-flat Netherlands, and the standard brakes they come equipped with are not suited to stopping at the bottom of a steep hill on a wet day with a full load of cargo. Brakes and gears should be altered to suit your terrain and weather.

The Bullitt, imported from Copenhagen, is another popular front loader option. It's lighter, and it handles more like a conventional bike. It isn't kid-ready out of the box the way a bakfiets is, but it is more flexible in its cargo capacity—it's ready to strap a carseat to or to fit seating (which you must make or buy separately) for a young passenger or two.

Cargo tricycles are another option for front loaders. Tricycles aren't for everyone, but a cargo trike has the advantage of always being upright when you are stopped—no need for a kickstand or to climb on and off at lights. The Box Bike and Nihola brands, both imported from Europe, are popular and increasingly available. A U.S. made option is the Haley Trike out of Philadelphia; being individually made, these are not necessarily cheaper but are more customizable, allowing for choices in the gearing and box shape.

As family bicycling becomes more popular, there are more and more front loaders on the market that are specifically designed for carrying kids.

Keeping kids happy on the bike

"It's okay to bribe them with treats. Then they sit on the bike and eat cookies instead of trying to take off their helmets." —Emily Finch, Portland, Oregon

"Having a word game makes it easy so that there is no time to complain. We would play word games like do the alphabet with bike related parts or items we see around us. My sons' favorite was each of us in turn taking turns adding to a story. Snacks also make it easy. It is hard to complain about being on a bike when dad has crackers, a bar, or apple slices." —Travis Wittwer, Portland

"The occasional trip in the car or on the bus is all it takes for me to appreciate how much easier the bike is. The two kids tend to argue in the car, but the moment we're on the bike, everything is joyful. We notice more exciting things—exciting to toddlers and preschoolers, that is—boats, train tracks, cement mixer trucks, etc." —Madeleine Carlson, Seattle

Always having snacks and water on hand for both you and the kids on your bike will significantly improve everyone's experience. Bringing toys and books along can also help keep your kid occupied in the trailer or bucket. If your child is a thrower, tie their toy or sippie cup down—try one of those spiral lanyards. Make sure it isn't long enough to get caught in a wheel when the item is chucked overboard.

Bikes that your kids ride with you
Tag-alongs

"I was surprised at how quickly they took to it and how much they enjoy it. Their enjoyment of riding is so obvious and so infectious that their 2 year old brother insists on a turn on the trail-a-bike too when it is out."
—Nicole Donnelly, Washington, DC (nieces aged 3 & 4)

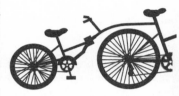

A tag-along is a single wheel, seat, and set of pedals that attaches to the back of your bike. Your child sits on the back and pedals—or doesn't. Like with a tandem, as the young pedaler grows stronger, they can really help power the bike uphill. Tag-alongs are loved by families of young kids who are able to bike on their own, but who can't necessarily go as far or fast as every trip requires. It's also good for kids who get restless sitting passively in a trailer.

When you drop your child off at school via a tag-along, you can remove it from your bike, lock it to a rack, and go about your day unemcumbered. Kids can start on these as soon as they're big enough to ride their own bike; the seats are adjustable so they can keep riding with them up to age eight or even older.

Tag-alongs are widely available used and in good condition. There are several varieties, with different attachments. Most attach to your seat post, which can interfere with your ability to use your rear rack; it can take a few minutes to get used to the feel of riding with one.

New and very popular is the Weehoo, which puts your child in a recumbent position, and a seat belt. Another option is the FollowMe, a device that connects your rear wheel with the front of your child's bike, producing the stable ride of a tandem, freeing up your rear rack,

It is possible to attach some kinds of bicycle trailer to the wheel of a tag-along to increase the capacity (and length!) of your family bike. Look at the weight rating on your tag-along before trying this, and heed it. Tag-along hitches have been known to suddenly fail when asked to exceed their recommended capacity.

Kid tandems

"Tandems are the most incredible things with kids. We'll set out for a short ride on the tandem, and she'll just sit back there telling me about absolutely everything in her world." —Kevin Turinsky, Anchorage, Alaska

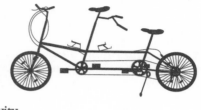

Tandem bikes are especially good for kids who are old enough to ride a bike but for whatever reason are not ready to independently ride their own bicycles everywhere. It's also a frequent and charming sight at longer rides to see parents and teens riding together on a tandem as a bonding activity.

There are a multitude of tandem bicycles out there that are meant to be piloted by an adult joined by either one or even two children. These bikes are not cheap, but they can be adjusted for growing kids and can be used for years.

In most of these the adult rides in the front, piloting the bike, while one or two children ride behind, stoking.

Newer types of family tandem allow the kid to ride in the front while the adult behind them maintains control over steering and braking. These bikes often are shorter than tandems (meaning the pilot in the rear can see around corners better than you might think) and at times resemble a hybrid between a tandem and a bike with a child's seat in the front, or a front loader where the passenger can pedal.

Kid tandems are typically designed so that the kid does not have to be pedaling for the bicycle to go forward—the adult can be doing all the work. Because these are similar to regular bicycles you can still put a rack and panniers over the front and rear wheels. Some parents will add on even more kids by putting a child seat over the rear wheel, or between them and the handlebars, or by towing a trailer or a tag-along behind.

A note on electric assists

Electric assists can be fitted to many cargo bike set-ups, and some specialty cargo bicycle shops also offer excellent electric assist options. Chapter 3 includes more details about the pros and cons of the electric assist. When it comes to family bicycling, some parents find an extra boost going up the hills they traverse regularly makes all the difference; others find the unit's battery to be heavy and bulky, one extra thing to carry and keep track of.

Shopping for family bikes

"For us, having the opportunity to test ride bicycles with the conditions we encounter daily would have been the greatest benefit. My five-minute test ride on the Yuba in Columbus, Ohio without my family is nothing like what we deal with adding moving weight and hills. When we were selecting a bicycle, we reached out to other bicycling families around the country and we are most happy we did. No one here had the information or the bicycles. It's been a lonely adventure in that respect, but one that has give us perspective and passion." —Stacy Bisker, Huntington, West Virginia

Family bicycling is still new to North America, which means that family bikes and gear can be expensive. Bikes and seats often need to be imported; locally made varieties tend to be manufactured in small quantities; either way the price can seem sky high.

Keep in mind that when it comes to cargo bikes you get what you pay for. If you're on a tight budget, look for a used bargain before you settle for a cheap knockoff. The good news is that the same factors that lead to high prices also mean that most cargo bikes on the market right now are so well made that even heavily used ones will often still be in great condition to meet your family's needs for many more years.

Buying a new cargo bikes can be the equivalent of investing in a used car, in both utility and price. But unlike a car, a utility bike needs to not just fit your passengers and stuff—it needs to fit you comfortably, as well as any other adults who will be piloting the bike. It also needs to have suitable gearing and brakes for the type of terrain you'll be riding on.

Test riding a bike before you purchase it is essential, especially if it is a pricey investment that you plan to use as a major family vehicle. That said, many families just read up about their options and jump in, and things work out well. Cargo bikes hold their value, and if your first attempt doesn't work out, another family will likely be very happy to take it off your hands.

If you live in a city that boasts a specialty cargo bike shop, then you're in luck. These shops tend to have small selections tended by knowledgeable and helpful owners. An increasing number of regular local bike shops carry one or more lines of cargo and kid-specific bikes. Ask at yours to see if they have anything for you to try. If not, you may need to get creative.

Another option is to find other early adopters near you who are willing to let you try their bikes out. If nobody in your town rides a bakfiets, maybe a family a few hours away has one. The Internet is a great resource for finding other bicycling families.

Another option is to go to where the bikes are. If you have a vacation or business travel planned to a city where there are bike shops that carry cargo bikes, then plan to test ride as many as you can during that time, preferably with your kids and something equivalent to a couple of bags of groceries on board. Some families plan their vacations specifically around this goal.

The appendix at *EverydayBicycling.com* includes a partial list of bike shops that specialize in cargo bikes, as well as links to the North American retailers of a long list of cargo bike brands.

Maintaining your cargo bike
While you seek out the bike setup of your dreams, conduct a simultaneous search for the mechanic of your dreams. The good news is that the more expensive the bike, the less maintenance it is likely to need. European imports are built to last forever with minimal care. The drivetrain is internal,

the tires are as durable and puncture proof as bike tires can be, and even the chain is enclosed in a case. This is a good thing, because they are extra difficult to work on and often require specially imported parts and tools.

Even if you don't need to take your bike in every month for a flat tire or squeaky brake, you will still need to do a tune-up once a year to keep the wheels spinning smoothly and the brakes stopping you safely. So unless you have a motivated handy person under your own roof, it's a good idea to start feeling out your local bike shops and seeing if one of them has a mechanic eager to take on the challenge of caring for your new ride.

Teaching your kids to ride independently
Balance bikes

Probably the best way—and definitely the cutest—to start your kid off learning to bicycle when they are tiny is with a balance bike, also called a scoot bike or a run bike. These resemble most of all the velocipedes of two hundred years ago—they have two wheels, handlebars and a seat, but no gears or pedals. The kid sits on the seat and propels themself forward with a running motion, also using their feet to stop. You walk or ride along with them, teaching them the fine art of stopping at intersections, looking for cars, and riding with others.

Learning to ride a balance bike tends to be the best way to prepare a child for the transition to a pedal bike. True to their name, they teach the most difficult part of bicycling—balance—in a way that tricycles and training wheels don't. If you have an older child who is learning to ride, or if you don't want to invest in a balance bike that will be quickly outgrown, you can get similar results, though with somewhat more ankle-bruising potential, by removing the pedals from the regular two wheeler your child will eventually ride. Once they are comfortable scooting and gliding around this way, put the pedals back on and they'll get the hang of it in no time.

Training wheels

Training wheels are still the standard way to start your kid out riding a bike. Here is how training wheels work: You install them on a two-wheeler so that they hover an inch off the ground when the bike is upright. The idea is that if the kid tips one way or the other, for instance while turning, the training wheel on that side can carry them for a minute until they are able to balance themselves upright again. Raise the wheels incrementally as the new bicyclist gains skills and confidence, until eventually they are no longer needed.

Training wheels are not an ideal solution for everyone. The most timid new cyclists tend to treat a bike mounted with training wheels as a tricycle, riding on three points—this does not help them learn balance or confidence and makes for an uncomfortable ride. If you are not having good luck with training wheels or would like to bypass them altogether, then for younger kids go with a balance bike, and for older kids and teens see the first chapter for tips on learning to ride.

Kids riding their own bikes

"I think the key is understanding the child, knowing when you need to go exactly at their pace and when it is ok to push just a little bit further. Kids like to say 'I can't' a lot. I have learned to ignore that and say 'but see, you just did' a lot. It is amazing how far a little encouragement goes." —Nicole Donnelly, Washington, DC

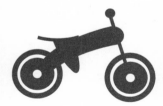

How old do you have to be to learn to ride? The answer varies, sometimes wildly—every kid learns at their own pace. Some are ready to roll as soon as they can toddle, while others aren't comfortable getting on a bike until they are in their teens or older.

You'll likely know when your own kids are ready. When that happens, how do you teach them to ride safely and confidently?

Teaching your kid to ride

Doug Smart in Corvallis teaches bike safety to school kids. Here are his guidelines:

- **Model expected behavior.** Kids aren't interested in things like formative vs. mature brains—if you expect them to wear their helmets, then you need to wear yours.

- **Consistency.** All the safety checks and behaviors need to be done the same way every time so they can become lifelong habits.

- **Responsibility.** For many kids bicycling is one of their first opportunities to interact with adults on a nearly equal basis. They are responsible for their own choices and the consequences of those choices to themselves and others.

- **Get comfortable!** If you're a nervous role model, your kids will learn to be nervous when they ride. This may mean doing family rides on off-street paths for a while as you both build skills.

- **Trust your kids**. Emphasize safety and offer some coaching and then shut up for a bit. Give them space to make mistakes.

- **Consider asking for help.** It is not abdicating parental responsibility to ask a friend to help out or to put your kids into a class to learn bike skills. Often kids will listen better to an adult who isn't their parent. Just make sure you and that other adult are reinforcing each other.

Riding together
Riding with your kid, especially when they're just starting out, will present a learning curve for you as well as for them.

Start with short rides, stopping while it's still fun, before your kid is tired or overwhelmed. Teach one or two new ideas at a time.

What you do is even more important than what you say. When riding with your kid, whether on separate bikes, or with them on the back of your bike, it's important to be confident and consistent. See Chapter 1 for basic skills and safety practices. If it is your habit to stop when it's necessary, signal your turns, hold your line, and know how to safely handle difficult traffic situations, then your kid will learn to ride safely without much instruction. Conversely, if you're a timid or aggressive rider, or if you treat stop signs differently when you're riding on your own, your kid will pick up on that and ride that way as well.

One question some parents have is where to ride in relation to their child. As with everything else, there's no right answer. Ride in front to control the pace, show the way, and ensure that the kid is going to stop. Ride behind to keep an eye on your kid, and protect their wiggle zone. If you say "stop" and the kid doesn't stop, you can zoom up ahead of them.

Choosing kids' bikes

"Nothing too complicated. Balance bikes are great for really small kids. Getting into grade school a standard bike with the pedals temporarily removed will serve the same purpose. A multi-speed bike is ok if they don't worry about shifting until they have the basics down. Beyond that, it needs to be something that can be easily adjusted to fit." —Doug Smart, Corvallis, Oregon

"If you're going to build your kid a bike, make one they'll want to be seen on." —Kevin Turinsky, Anchorage, Alaska

Every year it gets a little easier to find new bikes for kids. Go to a bike shop you trust and look for everything you would want on your own bike to make it comfortable for the type of riding your kid will be doing. Make sure it fits comfortably, and add fenders if your kid will be riding in wet weather, and a rack or basket for carrying things. Get them a helmet and a lock for the bike, and lights if they'll ever be riding at night.

There is a glut of cheaply assembled bicycles available at big box stores— these are tempting as an investment that will be quickly outgrown. But they are not designed to be ridden farther than the end of your driveway and even at such close range they tend to fall apart quickly. Buying a kids' bike from a local bike shop will help ensure a higher level of both quality and service as your child begins their independent bicycling life.

Another good option is to go vintage. Most bikes used to be built to last. Your chances of finding an old banana seat cruiser in good condition will go up considerably the less popular bicycling is where you live. You'll need to get any vintage bike thoroughly tuned up and you may need to replace all the rubber before it's road ready, but this can be an attractive and relatively affordable option.

Used bikes of a more recent era are also often a good option. If your kid doesn't have an older sibling to inherit an outgrown bicycle from, perhaps a friend or neighbor is ready to move on. Also, community bike projects or co-ops often have a surplus of kid's bikes available to build up.

Kids grow, and it's safe to assume that most kids' bikes won't be with you for long, which is another reason to invest in a good quality one that you'll be able to resell.

At the same time, make sure that the bicycle you choose doesn't have too much room to grow. Trying to balance on a bike is tricky enough, and it's even harder when you have trouble reaching the pedals, much less the ground.

A final option for kids once they get into grade school is folding bikes. The seatpost and reach are fairly adjustable, though length tends to be a bit more of an issue. If a kid is reaching too far, they'll have trouble controlling the bicycle. But once your child is able to comfortably ride a folding bicycle, they'll be able to keep the same bike through adulthood.

Family biking logistics
Safety
Safety is a relative concept, and deeply disputed. It's hard to shake the idea that cars are safe, and this feeling of safety has led to something of an arms race in the size and weight of family vehicles. But statistically speaking, children are in more imminent physical danger while in and around motor vehicles than in any other situation. And the lasting effects of inactivity and social isolation are even greater in children than in adults.

In reality, we each have a different threshold when it comes to what feels safe and what doesn't. And whatever your theories about safety, the reality of the roads on which you travel will likely have an even greater impact on your decisions about bicycling. Here are just a few perspectives:

"We have found most every town can be traversed by bicycle. It is a matter of knowing where to go, being flexible, having an understanding of your community and its life pattern. We are familiar with which streets have more car traffic, where to go at night for better lighting, less pot holes or where the sidewalk may be the favorable and safer location. All of this has taken time and practice. There are places we would not travel by bicycle with our children, but would go there alone or with other adults. Our children can be more unpredictable on a bicycle and some roads require a lot more attention. Some places are too far for their endurance. Sometimes we travel late at night and we prefer to know we can get everyone home without them falling asleep at the handlebar." —Stacy Bisker, Huntington, West Virginia

"I think safety has to come first when you are taking a child with you, and that can be an absolute deal breaker. We lived in central Texas until Cora was one year old, and cycling with her was completely out of the question. The issue was cultural as much as it was about infrastructure. This was one of many factors in our decision to relocate to a place like Portland. It's completely different here. Getting started was so easy. Now the challenge is choosing to get out there in the rain and dark whenever we can with her. Honestly, the car is always there as a backup" —Chris Trahey, Portland (kid aged 2.5)

"It took Tyler a little while to get used to wearing a helmet, but we made it clear it was necessary and now he doesn't even think twice about wearing it." —Kristi Wood, Anchorage, Alaska

"We have to assume that we are completely invisible and most of the time it seems like we are." —Sarah Noga, Arlington, Washington

"Have belief that kids will be safe and that a parent has the skill to keep them safe. Routes should be planned; riding in traffic should be taught and practiced; and riding on a street involves a level of focus that is different than riding on a sidewalk." —Travis Wittwer, Portland

Weather

"Many parents seem to think children are fragile humans that must be sheltered from the elements, when in our opinion, as long as you dress your child appropriately, there is no reason to shield them from inclement weather. We think it's good for kids to learn how to be comfortable and enjoy themselves in 'bad' weather." —Kristi Wood, Anchorage, Alaska

"We don't go out with children in heavy rain. We go out in light to moderate rain when we must, and we go out prepared. Clothing has certainly been something we have been investing in. All the children now have waterproof jackets. We haven't bothered with waterproof pants yet, but use snow pants in colder weather." —Stacy Bisker, Huntington, West Virginia

A number of parents have confided to me that Portland's incessant rain seems to bother them far more than their kids; several said their kids actually love to ride in the rain.

The same weather advice given for adult riders in Chapter 2 applies to young ones. Drink a lot of water and play it safe in very hot weather; when it's cold or rainy, focus primarily on staying warm rather than staying dry.

Fenders are a must when you have kids on your bike in wet weather, or in a trailer or tagalong behind you. Rain and/or sun covers can be purchased for many cargo bikes, and are well worth the extra investment. Bring a towel to wipe off bike seats that have gotten wet while the bike is parked. Kids who are sitting still on a bike will get colder than ones pedaling, and need warmer clothes; but impermeable rain gear is less likely to be a problem. Waterproof ponchos with hoods are good raincoats for growing kids, and can be draped over the bike seat along with the kid to keep water from pooling below them; a drawstring sewn into the bottom hem can prevent it from blowing around.

Life logistics and scheduling
"The flattest route is always better than the shortest route."
—Emily Finch, Portland, Oregon

"We have to plan out grocery stops better and do less of the 'I forgot one thing let me drive back to the store and get it' kind of impulsive trips. Uh, yeah...we get to eat a lot more, too." —Sarah Noga, Arlington, Washington

"One trick is to encourage play dates that are close to our house, so that we have less distance to go." —Kristi Wood, Anchorage, Alaska

"I need to get over my tendency to apologize for having to schedule around the extra time it sometimes takes to arrive by bike." —Madeleine Carlson, Seattle

"We have tried hard to not replace many of our former auto destinations, enjoyments, or habits but found that we do end up declining some party invitations because of distance, or not running out for plumbing parts 17 miles away. We have learned to prioritize our time and energy, something we had previously been on the track to do, but increased our conscientious efforts with this transition. We may drive to a far away party, but it is because the host is a good friend, not just because we received a classmate invitation. We once waited three days for the local hardware store to open and made do with just one working toilet. In either situation, there were only benefits to be found." —Stacy Bisker, Huntington, West Virginia

The pace of life changes by bicycle; and this becomes even more true once you have kids. Getting kids out the door no matter what vehicle you use can be a challenge; by bicycle it can become more time consuming, when extra things like rain gear and helmets need to be found and adjusted. Bicycling outside of the neighborhood also tends to take longer when you're carrying kids.

Logistical issues result in many bicycling families simply going fewer places and partaking in fewer extracurricular activities. For many parents and their kids, this is a net positive, resulting in less time on the go and more time and freedom to play.

Bicycling families often—though by no means always—include one parent who works from home or part time, or a parent whose full time job is child rearing. This arrangement is frequently made more financially feasible by the choice to sell a car or drive it less.

Creating community

"If there are local biking groups, go on a group ride. Kidical Mass rides are wonderful to ride with...or just meet them at their end point if you're not ready to climb aboard your bike just yet. But many cities have group rides that aren't specifically family-oriented, but are geared towards new riders or riders of all abilities. Seeing real people out there is great, but it's also inspiring to connect with other biking parents online: read blogs, tweets, join Facebook groups, whatever it takes to see that people out there are getting out there every day—and we'd love to have you join us!" —Madeleine Carlson, Seattle

"Find opportunities wherever you are, as close to home as possible, and just start riding. If you feel that the community or infrastructure is a roadblock to safe and fun cycling, consider what it says about the community and then do one of two things: become the champion of change or relocate." —Chris Trahey, Portland

"If you're not already, get active in every aspect of transportation and development planning in your community that you can. The earlier the better. This will allow you to have a positive and beneficial impact on your transportation choices and options, as well as allow your children to see how the process works and how to improve it." —Kevin Turinsky, Anchorage, Alaska

"Joining a local Kidical Mass ride or creating your own weekend ride with other interested families is a great way to both create community as well as learn from each other." —Travis Wittwer, Portland

Meeting other bicycling families often leads to opportunities to socialize at your own pedal-powered pace, as well as to share information, resources, and to get involved in improving bicycling conditions in your community. There are any number of ways to connect with other families; two of the most successful in recent years are Kidical Mass and Bike Trains.

Kidical Mass has sprung up in the last several years and happens in cities all over the country. It's a short, slow-paced ride, in which families with kids of all ages and skills, on all kinds of bikes, ride together in the street. Usually these rides are short, stick to relatively low-traffic streets, and involve a park on one end and an ice cream shop on the other. Anybody can organize a Kidical Mass ride—see tips in Chapter 6. Like its namesake, Critical Mass, it's a lot of fun as well as being a valuable venue to meet other families and start to get comfortable riding in the street.

"Bike trains and bike buses are useful. When I took the kids to school via bike, we went about half of the time with a bike bus. It made our numbers larger so we were a better presence on the road and provided a sense of community; connecting my sons with other capable adults." —Travis Wittwer, Portland

Bike trains and walking school buses aren't a new idea, but they're enjoying a surge in popularity as a way for kids to walk and bike to school with adult supervision and safety in numbers. Sometimes they're organized by local college students, other times parents or school volunteers take turns leading as many as a hundred kids by bike through neighborhood streets to school. They tend to meet at a park and make their way to school through back streets, sometimes stopping to pick up more kids along the way. A good number of adults are on hand to help out wobbly riders, ensure safety, and cheer on the young participants.

More tips
A single chapter can hardly encapsulate all there is to say about family bicycling. The topic demands its own book—until that can be written, I'll leave you with these wise words of advice from our experts:

"80% of bike commuting is above the shoulders. It's developing the mind-set that overcomes all the little excuses that tend to keep us from doing new things." —Kristi Wood, Anchorage, Alaska

"We get lots of questions and inquiries on just about every trip. I feel this is my opportunity to demystify our car-free lifestyle." —Sarah Noga, Arlington, Washington

"Kickstands get treated as an 'accessory' but with family bikes, they really ought to be standard, and sturdy, and ideally, two-footed. Kids will climb around on bikes." —Katie Proctor, Portland, Oregon (kids ages 1 and 3)

"Bells. Kids love a good bell and the giving of a bell can be a token of accomplishment—you have done great and are ready for having a bell for when we ride in the street. And correctly adjusted helmets. Low on the forehead." —Travis Wittwer, Portland

"Make it special. My nieces and I have matching bike bracelets and matching bike tee shirts and we call ourselves a girl bike gang. Boys can ride with us, but they can't join! We don't always wear them, but it is something we have that creates more of a bond." —Nicole Donnelly, Washington, DC

"Families with special needs can do this too!" —Kathleen Youell, Portland, Oregon (kids aged 5 and 7)

"Start young and tell your kids why you prefer cycling. Get the right gear and consider moving to a neighborhood that is conducive to walking and cycling. The rent may be higher but it will save you money in the long run, increase your quality of life, and lower your worry factor." —Dan and Kirsten Kaufman, Portland, Oregon

"Just start slow and get out there!" —Madeleine Carlson, Seattle

6

Get organized!

The first bike event I organized was terrifying. It was a cold November night and I was absolutely certain both that nobody would show up and that a large crowd would be there looking to me for direction. I put off leaving minute by minute, unnecessarily re-reading the organizing and publicity emails, counting the homemade signs rolled in a tube in my bike basket, wondering if the nausea I suddenly felt was a good enough excuse to stay home.

But finally I forced myself to go, rolling up to the meeting point ten minutes late. My second-greatest fear had come true—there was a sizeable crowd, two reporters with notebooks, and a film crew in an SUV, all looking at me expectantly. Within minutes, I had made several new friends, given my first television interview, and was on my bike, happily doing the thing I love most—riding through Portland's streets with a crew of chatting, cheery fellow riders.

The goal of the ride wasn't the same for everyone there. Some wanted to raise awareness about inconsistent police enforcement of bicycle laws. Others wanted to send a message to cyclists to stop at every stop sign, and yet others wanted to send the same message to car drivers. For many of us, getting together to ride, meeting other riders, and talking about cycling was the underlying objective. We didn't have to agree on the issue at hand in order to want to make sure the public conversation about bicycling reflected the complexities that we encountered every day on the road.

Bikes and community

Bicycling can be empowering and transformative on a purely personal level. But it can also get a bit lonely, especially if you live somewhere it hasn't caught on yet. When you're out there alone, indignities tend to pile on: hostile drivers, misinformed police officers, unsafe streets and dangerous road crossings. Some people handle these difficulties by moving—across town, or perhaps even to a new city or country. Many others stay right where they are and work to improve bicycling conditions—much to the benefit of many a place that ten years ago would not have been seen as a likely bike-friendly community.

Many riders quickly discover the value of riding with others. Having a friend, coworker, or spouse to ride with, or even just to talk with about riding, is one of the primary factors that helps people start riding and keep it up. Having several friends, or a community, is what turns cycling into a way of life and allows it to become a widespread movement.

Subcultures are constantly emerging around bikes. You're probably already familiar with the sight of lycra'd out recreational riders pedaling around back country roads on a sunny weekend. Then there are the lawyers who go on hard and fast competitive lunchtime rides. Messengers get together and hold urban alleycat races. Grassroots bike festivals bring people together in cities around the world for purposes as wide-ranging as bike commuter breakfasts, educational sightseeing tours, and political protests. Critical Mass, though controversial, has served an essential function as an incubator for many bicycle organizations and events with more mainstream appeal. Cultures rise up around bike polo, welding and riding tall bikes, bicycle dance, riding restored vintage bikes, bicycle-themed art, teen bike programs, and anything else you can imagine.

Riding in a group allows you to check out what kind of bikes other people are riding, what they wear when they ride, what routes they take, how they handle turns and stops and hills, and to compare notes and share resources. Even if you're the only person you know who rides a bike, the Internet can be a huge boon in the same way. There are many online forums where the smallest topics in cycling are discussed and argued about to an absurd—and extremely helpful—level of detail.

The value of building bicycle community is substantial on several levels. Being around other riders—on the roads, in the office, at the bar or coffeeshop, or online—is validation. Especially if you're a pioneer, as a transportation cyclist, or riding with kids, or riding at all, you will benefit greatly from regular reminders that you aren't the only one, that your choice to ride is sane and relatively safe one, that you aren't blocking traffic, and that someday in the not-so-distant future you might have a lot of two-wheeled company.

Getting organized
Beginning to ride a bike has been the occasion for many an ordinary citizen to become a dedicated attendee of city council meetings, documenter of road conditions, and amateur urban planning expert. The effects of these efforts are palpable, and usually of great benefit to the surrounding community, bike riders and otherwise. As you learn, don't forget to talk—and listen—to others. You can do a lot on your own, but your advocacy will have a more lasting impact when it clearly comes from the community.

Starting a group
Maybe you want to do more than just go on one bike ride. Maybe you'd like to start a group that meets regularly and can discuss issues online as well. Forming a group is a powerful tool for tapping into the energy in your community for improving bicycling conditions, or just to meet other people who ride bikes.

The old fashioned way
It used to be that if you wanted to get a group of people together who share a passion for the same issue or cause, you would reach them by leaving fliers at places they were likely to spend time.

Even in the age of the Internet, this method still works—and sometimes works even better than a social media campaign. If you want to hold a meeting to talk about a local intersection that's dangerous for cycling or to start a social riding group, it's easy to create and photocopy an invitation and post it in bike shops, coffee shops, offices, student unions, on bike parking racks, and anywhere else where a rider or potentially interested person might see them. Then show up at the appointed time and place prepared with paper and pens so you can take notes and gather everyone's contact information.

If only one other person shows up, you've got the seeds of something real. If you get three or more attendees, congratulation: you have a movement.

If you are holding a meeting about a particular issue and are concerned that someone will come who opposes your effort and wants to derail it, make sure you have your allies and arguments lined up ahead of time. But don't forget to listen to your project's opponents, too; their concerns are likely valid, and your efforts will be all the stronger if you can find a way to work together.

Blogs
Have a way with words, or with computers? Are you inclined to observe, listen, and report? There's a real niche out there for bicycle blogging. The most successful blogs are either hyper-local, reporting on the details of roads, issues, events, and people in a particular region, city, or even neighborhood. Other bloggers choose a topical niche, such as vintage bicycles, biking with children, or analyzing legal issues in bicycling, and are able to find an audience and make their mark in that way.

Setting up a website is easy, and can be as simple as signing up for a free site through Blogger or Wordpress. Gaining an audience requires more work and requires regularly producing topical, readable content, reaching out to potential readers and to other writers and businesses that serve them, and finding a rhythm that doesn't burn out you, the blogger.

Established bloggers often are able to increase the amount of time they dedicate to the blogs by monetizing them. The bike bloggers most successful at earning a living from their work tend to be ones who have created an essential community resource that provides readers with opportunities to connect with each other and tap into broader happenings in the blogger's chosen realm.

Forums and lists

Plain old email lists, where you hit "reply-all" can get unwieldy quickly once you have more than three or four people involved. Email groups and lists, meetup groups, or listservs, are the next step up; they're centrally organized, people can choose to add and remove themselves, and a moderator can ensure that things run smoothly and spam doesn't take over.

Forums are similar, but instead of every message being delivered to every member's inbox, participants must actively go to the forum's page and look at what others' have posted. Forums are excellent when more people are involved and working on diverse projects or discussing diverse interests that don't necessarily overlap.

Both forums and listservs are excellent when there's a community of people in a similar area or with a niche interest who want to have regular interactions or ongoing conversation. These are great organizing tools for changeling may peoples' energy into a project or into discussing issues. People can share their research, ideas and information spontaneously. They can also propose and begin organizing rides and events. They can also toss around proposals, ideas and keep each other inspired/encouraged/motivated. These are especially great when their members can also get together in person regularly, though it doesn't have to be that way.

Meetings

If at all possible, it's always better to get people together in person, even if not frequently, on a regular basis. Whether you are planning an event, brainstorming a lobbying session, founding a new organization or just having a social event over beer/hot chocolate, meeting up in person is important. This is where having a listserve, server, or blog comes in handy because it can get people together and then allow people who were unable to meet to see all of the info discussed in the event displayed in one place.

Meetings are where the best schemes happen. Make sure everyone has a chance to introduce themselves and share their ideas. Don't forget to make the meeting fun. Go for a ride afterwards.

Unless your meetings are merely social, don't have them for "no reason." It helps to have a facilitator *and* a note-taker who can then put notes online or otherwise share them with the group.

How to lead a ride

Leading a bike ride can be done for fun, to meet people, for a political purpose, or just to ride. Everyone on the ride doesn't need to share the same motivation. A ride can be a great way to get people together, build community, and get a different feeling for the streets of your community. You can safely ride on streets you would not necessarily brave on your own.

Step one: Choose a theme or a purpose for your ride. Are you riding to a destination, like a coffee shop, bar, a movie or to testify at city hall? Or is the purpose of your ride to explore nearby trails, learn about local history, or see bike infrastructure? You could also have a ride for a social reason—like to get together with other people who have cargo bikes, host a singles ride, or just for fun among friends.

Step two: Chose a date and time for the ride. Make sure it doesn't conflict with the date and time of another event your riders may be interested in joining. If it does, see if you can start/end at the same location. Also choose a starting location. If it's a business or public gathering place, call ahead to make sure they'll open and as a courtesy to let them know there might be a rush.

Step three: Plan your route. Ride your route in advance. Tailor the route (such as which streets it goes down) depending on your participants. Is it an "in your face" ride to go down main streets to make a statement, or is it a social ride for little kids to get ice-cream and ding their bells? Scout out your route again a day or two before the actual ride to make sure there is no construction or other obstacles have popped up. It's good to know what turns/intersections you'll go through and whether or not you'll need ride helpers. Sometimes it's nice and safer to have people block intersections on larger rides.

Step four: Promote your ride. Make a flier, promote it on the internet, send it out over email lists, tell your friends, ask organizations to spread the word, or you could even send out a press release. It's an obvious thing to say, but people often forget to mention vital information on posters and in emails. Make sure you include: name, date, starting time, starting place, ending place, phone number and any other information people need to know (like who is the ride appropriate for?)

If you want the info to show up in newspapers/calendars, you may need to let them know a month in advance. For tv, radio and blogs, let reporters know at least a week in advance and give them a reminder the day before. Of course if you are not planning your ride to be very big, you may not need to do all of this, but even if you want just 10 people to come, you'll need to make sure they have all of the information.

Step five: The ride itself. Arrive at the meeting place early. It'll be your job to make sure the ride leaves more or less on time. You may want to leave 5-10 minutes after the announced start time to allow stragglers to join you, but any longer than that and people get restless. For a ride of more than a dozen or so people, it's a good idea to have one person leading the pack and at least one other person who knows the route who can bring up the rear in case someone gets a flat tire or is otherwise going slowly. If the group gets split up by red lights or flat tires, make sure the people at the front know that is happening, so they can wait for everyone else. Unless it's a race, keep it slow! There's a big difference between recreational rides for fitness and social rides for exploration, chatting, or protest.

Step six: After the ride, thank everyone for coming. If there's a good feeling and people want to keep hanging out, head to a bar or coffee shop. Start planning the next step!

Step seven: Follow up. Set a date for any follow-up activities, the next ride, or meeting and let participants know about it. Add new folks to the email list or let them know where they can find more information, and make sure they have a way to contact each other. If any members of the media covered your event, be sure to thank them.

Advocacy
If you are inclined to love diplomatic endeavors and untangling complex technical details, you might be a born advocate.

If you have a local bicycle or active transportation advocacy organization, contact them to find out how to get involved. Most offer basic volunteer opportunities like stuffing envelopes, or staffing the registration table at fundraising rides. These are great ways to get to know an organization, see how and if you might fit in to higher level volunteer positions, or see opportunities for new advocacy that their organization does not address. Depending on your skills and interests, you might end up helping organize events, monitoring legislative hearings, drafting position papers, or sitting on a committee dedicated to fundraising, outreach, or strategic planning.

If there is no local organization whose work appeals to you, consider starting one. Even if you are not so inclined, you can still be an effective advocate on your own by testifying at City Hall, writing a letter to the editor, lobbying your state (or national) representatives, getting signatures for voter referendums, or even running for office yourself.

Approaching city hall
Sometimes city hall is ready to help you; the powers that be just may not yet realize there is a need. In other cases, there may be obstructions. Your approach will depend on your local political climate, who is responsible for creating safer conditions for bicycling, and how receptive they are to actually doing so.

Sometimes advocacy can be as simple as a phone call or letter. If there is a major pothole on your bike route, glass in the bike lane on a major street, or an intersection along your route where people in cars routinely run the red light, you can call and report it; look online or in the blue pages for the proper number. If your request is fulfilled, be sure to write a thank you note.

If you have a more complicated project, or if repeated requests haven't been effective, it's time to get organized.

Your first step is to decide what to ask for. Perhaps it's a bike lane on a busy road that is about to be repaved—this is an excellent time to make infrastructure changes because the cost of re-striping the road already needs to be spent. Other potential asks include lowering the speed limit on a street near a school, having bike parking installed in front of the library, hosting a ciclovia-style open streets event, or dedicating a certain percentage of the transportation budget to bicycling infrastructure.

Your next step is to do the research and talk to the stakeholders. Familiarize yourself with local laws. Perhaps your city has a transportation plan or even a bicycle master plan. Try to meet with the mayor or the person on the city council in charge of transportation, with the city-employed transportation planner in charge of bicycling infrastructure, and with any business owners, residents, or other people who might be affected by or have a direct interest in this project.

This is not the time to make demands, but rather to build relationships. From these conversations, you will gain helpful contacts and get a sense of who will be an ally and in what capacity. You may also find that you need to change what you are asking for. For instance, maybe there isn't room for a bike rack in front of the library, but the owners of the pharmacy next door have the extra sidewalk width and wouldn't be opposed to a rack so long as they don't have the responsibility of maintaining it.

Your next step is to decide how to go forward. Often, your meeting with the mayor may be all that is necessary—or you might need to write them a detailed follow up letter. Don't underestimate the value of a well-researched letter to city hall, showing a need for a project and describing how it will improve the city while being cost-effective. You can also often make progress by testifying at city hall—extra points if you have business owners and other advocates lined up to give their testimony as well.

Politicians don't like to do anything without knowing that that they have citizen backup, and that the project will gain them more goodwill than criticism.

For that reason, among others, it is above all important to have, and prove, the support of the community for the project. To do this you need to actually make sure community members back you up. Listen very carefully to anyone who does not support or agree with you. If you can adjust your project or rhetoric to meet their needs, they might become allies instead of opponents. Even if this is not possible, you will likely have a good deal to learn from them.

Then, keep following up until the changes are made. Quite a bit of persistence is often necessary. If you run into roadblocks—either active opposition or simple inaction—don't give up. See the next section for more ways to demonstrate public support.

All of this is also true at the state and federal level. All you can do is learn everything you can, keep talking to people, keep your issue in the public eye, and persist until you make it. This may involve lawsuits, or trips to the capitol, or even launching major political campaigns—but those are all-consuming endeavors. Start small and you might be amazed by what you can accomplish.

Advocacy case study
In Missoula, Montana a guy named Bob runs the city's community bicycle project and also serves as the town's main bike, transit, and walking advocate, regularly visiting city hall to weigh in on planned bicycle improvements (or lack thereof). One day, Bob went out to meet the road crew that was about to start painting a new bike lane on a major street. Their plan called for a four foot wide bike lane. Bob told them that five feet is recognized as the preferred width for a safe and comfortable lane. After hearing him out, the crew moved their machine over a foot and painted the new white stripes five feet apart.

Bikes and party politics
Bicycle transportation is one of those rare issues that has appeal across all party lines. Liberals and conservatives can agree on the values of improving conditions for bicycling. Conservatives might be more inclined to point out the huge cost of our existing road system and the substantial economic savings, both individual and societal, as incentives to choose bicycling. Liberals might focus instead on the health, social, and environmental rewards

of encouraging people to bike instead of drive. All points can potentially be agreed upon across the board. If you're lucky, you live somewhere that bicycling has not become politically polarized. Otherwise, the best you can do is argue the case for bicycling on its merits and not play into the partisan arguments.

Bikes at work

While many employers go out of their way to encourage employees to bike to work, many others are less inclined to provide material support such as secure parking out of the elements or places to shower and change after a long ride in. A few employers will even attempt to prevent their employees from riding.

If your employer doesn't encourage or actively discourages bicycling, it might be enough simply to ask for a change. On your own time, research bicycle parking costs and feasibility and present the plan to management. It might help to demonstrate the financial benefits that come from freeing up another car parking space, and presenting research about the benefits to employers in health care costs and productivity that stem from promoting active commutes.

If there are other bicycle commuters at your workplace, consider starting or joining a friendly competition to log bike commute days or miles within the company or between different businesses. Building a culture of cycling will eventually make the case and create the demand for bigger changes in the workplace.

Getting business on board

As you work to improve your city for bicycling, you'll find that local businesses large and small are among your strongest allies and your fiercest opponents.

When business owners, managers, and staff go out of their way to support cycling, even in small ways, let them know you appreciate it. Like politicians, business owners are much more likely to hear complaints than praise, and will often respond strongly to thanks—especially when those accolades are paired with an increase in visibility or customers.

Despite increasing evidence that cycling and walking customers tend to spend more than driving ones at downtown retail locations, many business owners are still skeptical of anything bicycle-related. Even the most anti-bike ones can often be won over, though. In these cases money may talk better than actual arguments. If a retail business is resisting bicycle facilities on their street, organize a ride with the purpose of visiting their business and spending money. Or ask everyone you know to go patronize the business, helmet in hand and ask the owner to support the bicycle improvements.

Sometimes a business owner might simply not be aware of cyclists' needs or that they are being friendly or unfriendly to them. For instance, if a delivery truck regularly parks in the bike lane outside a store, or the bike rack area is used to display merchandise, all you might need is a friendly letter to the owner letting them know that you support their business but need to have a safe and convenient way to bike there.

Bikes in the Media

When bicycle transportation makes it into the media, it isn't always in a positive light. We've all probably

Business case study

In Portland, Oregon, the city's transportation department deployed a successful campaign to improve bike parking citywide. For years, a small bike parking fund has been available to install a bike staple that parks two bikes in the space between sidewalk and street for any business that requested it. The demand for bike parking had grown larger than these staples could accommodate, though, and some businesses were starting to demand more.

So the city set up a program to build "bike corrals," which replace one or two on-street car parking spots with between ten and twenty bike parking spaces. City transportation leaders signed up four prominent local businesses to test the program. When the plan was announced, there was considerable pushback from other business owners—losing car parking meant losing money, they declared.

The corrals went in and quickly filled with bikes. The initial businesses suddenly had more convenient parking spaces for paying customers, and other businesses almost immediately started demanding their own bike corrals. One restaurant owner started a petition. Now there are over 70 bike corrals throughout the city, with a long waiting list for more. Cities around the country are finding that installing bike corrals is one of the most affordable and politically feasible ways to encourage bicycling and give a boost to the local economy.

read at least one story in the local newspaper, or seen one on TV, covering a new bike lane, a bike event, or a crash in a way that doesn't seem to fairly portray cycling in general or a particular cyclist.

The good news is that as bicycling becomes more popular as a way to get around, media professionals are taking it up as well. But even if an individual reporter does ride a bike, their editor might not be bike-friendly—or a reporter in a hurry might just pull a story about a crash directly from the police reports, or a story about bicycle funding directly from a highway lobby press release.

It behooves bicycle riders to be alert and media savvy in framing and responding to stories. When you're talking about bikes to the media, remember that you are telling a story more or less directly to people in your community. Imagine how you would talk about your cause to someone you know and respect, and tell the story that way.

Pitching reporters
One way to get realistic, positive stories about bicycle transportation in the news is to be proactive. Anyone can contact a reporter and suggest a story. Maybe you have an event, ride, or issue to publicize. If not, think about the most inspiring bicycle story you know. For instance, is your workplace or a local business especially friendly to bicycling? Or you can suggest yourself as a subject, focusing on how you work bicycle transportation into your life. This story will be most appealing if bicycling is unusual where you live, or if you do something outside the norm—for example, running a business by bike, biking with kids, commuting long distances, or carrying things that most people would assume requires a car.

Reporters will be more likely to cover your story if you make their job easier by giving them everything they need up front in a pitch. This includes a narrative for the story itself, which will preferably provide either an element of surprise, conflict, or overcoming obstacles. You'll also want to tell the reporter why their particular audience would be interested in the story and, if relevant, what section of their publication the story would be good for. Anything else you can provide that will help make the story quick and easy will make it that much more likely to happen—send quotations and photos to a blogger or newspaper writer; let a TV or radio editor know about strong visual or audio elements.

Then compile your pitch into an email of no more than three or four short paragraphs. Take some care with the wording; a hurried news outlet may simply copy and paste your words. Be sure to include your contact information as well as any necessary details about dates, times, and locations. If you aren't sure who to send your pitch to, call or email the news outlet with a quick question, like: "Who do I send a pitch about a family of six that gets around by bicycle?" If you are pitching multiple outlets, personalize each pitch and send them individually. When someone bites, get back to them quickly. Even if you don't hear a response, it's fine to send a follow-up email or reminder a week later.

Working with the media is all about developing relationships. When a reporter writes a story based on your pitch, thank them for their coverage. If you liked the way the story turned out, be sure to put them at the top of your list when you pitch future stories. Likewise, be sure to thank reporters and editors for any positive coverage of bicycling, especially if that isn't standard.

Responding to stories
When you see a story that seems unfairly negative or biased towards bicycling, there are several ways to respond.

If a basic fact is wrong, you can request a correction from the paper. If a major perspective in a story isn't represented, you can contact the reporter directly to fill in the gaps and let them know that there's more to the story than they might have initially uncovered. If you are friendly and provide good, concise information, the reporter might just call you up in advance the next time they are assigned a story about cycling.

You can also respond to a story, positive or negative, by writing a letter to the editor or leaving a comment on the online version of the story. When crafting these, it is best to be brief, informative, and levelheaded. Write a couple of drafts and let the final one sit for a while before posting or sending it. Make sure your facts are impeccable and your tone is confident and encouraging.

Remember that any time you speak or write publicly about bicycling, you will reach a large audience of people—including reporters and editors themselves—who may be hostile or uninformed about cycling now, but who have the potential to become sympathetic allies, and who are likely to start cycling themselves one day and forget that they ever thought of it as anything other than a joyful experience.

Conclusion

I was timid and tentative about cycling for many years. I didn't start to feel truly comfortable on a bike in traffic until I started spending time with other people who rode bikes every day. My new bike friends and I would ride through the city at night in search of empty streets and late donuts, debate stop signs and turn signals, argue over our favorite places to cross the interstate or get up the ridge in the northeast part of town, and egg each other on to organize events or write letters to city hall.

Bicycling became a mark of pride for me, of identity and community. Being a cyclist meant I stopped riding the bus and no longer begged for rides from friends. I began to apply for bike-related jobs, go on bicycle dates, write long op-eds about bicycle laws, infrastructure, and culture, and dedicate myself to learning about cycling and being a bicycle activist in every spare moment of every day. I started to think of myself as a bicyclist.

I also started to notice that a few old friends also rode bikes all the time. I invited one of them to a group ride I was participating in, something silly involving costumes. She wasn't interested. "I don't want to be a cyclist," she said. "I just want to ride my bike to the grocery store."

For cycling advocates, this attitude is the ideal end goal: That getting around by bicycle becomes so normal that everyone can just get on a bike every day without thinking twice about it, and without changing their habits or identity, or needing to read a book like this one.

My dream is that within the next decade this book, along with the idea of identifying as a cyclist, will be obsolete, a curiosity. I hope that someday soon all young children will learn to ride, and that bicycling will become so normal that nobody has to think twice about it. I love the passion of my bicycle communities, but I envision the day when that energy and creativity can be directed elsewhere. That cultural shift is already happening, and by reading this book you are a part of it.

Now get out there and ride your bike!

Acknowledgments

This book owes all of its merit to the many, many people I've talked with and learned from about bicycling over the years, and particularly to the generous souls who shared their knowledge and ideas during the writing process of this book. All errors and omissions are purely my own.

The family bicycling chapter owes its existence to the smarts of friends and strangers. Special thanks to Katie Proctor for reviewing a rough draft and making helpful suggestions, and to Kath Youell, Emily Finch, Kevin Turinsky, Nicole Donnelly, Chris Trahey, Travis Wittwer, Kristi Wood, Dan and Kirsten Kaufman, Doug Smart, Eric Moody, Madeleine Carlson, Stacy Bisker, Kathleen Youell, and Sarah Noga for telling me their stories and lending their words to the text.

Caroline Paquette read two chapters in draft form and, once she stopped laughing, provided vital technical revisions. Sara Stout mused spontaneously and productively about a range of topics I always had to rush to write down. Erik Sandblom, Lisa Finn, and Austin Horse lent their wisdom about some of the more vital myriad details.

Kate Berube and Meghan Sinnott typed several large chunks of the manuscript. Davey Oil did the dishes and maintained much-needed good cheer during the final two weeks of writing.

Joe Biel listened to every detail and believed in me every day, and is the best partner you could ever hope for in hauling an unbelievable amount of scrap lumber across town, and in everything else.

SUBSCRIBE TO EVERYTHING WE PUBLISH!

Do you love what Microcosm publishes?

Do you want us to publish more great stuff?

Would you like to receive each new title as it's published?

Subscribe as a BFF to our new titles and we'll mail them all to you as they are released!

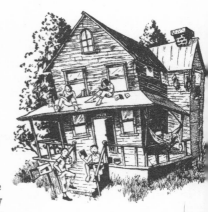

$10-30/mo, pay what you can afford. Include your t-shirt size and month/date of birthday for a possible surprise! Subscription begins the month after it is purchased.

microcosmpublishing.com/bff